THE TRUST PRESCRIPTION FOR HEALTHCARE

Building Your Reputation with Consumers

THE TRUST PRESCRIPTION FOR HEALTHCARE

Building Your Reputation with Consumers

David A. Shore

Health Administration Press
Chicago, IL

Your board, staff, or clients may also benefit from this book's insight. For more information on quantity discounts, contact the Health Administration Press Marketing Manager at (312) 424-9470.

09 08 5 4

Library of Congress Cataloging-in-Publication Data here

Shore, David.

The trust prescription for healthcare: building your reputation with consumers/ David A. Shore.

p. : cm.

Includes bibliographical references.

ISBN-10: 1-56793-240-1

ISBN-13: 978-1-56793-240-9

1. Medical care—Public opinion. 2. Patient satisfaction. 3. Consumer education. 4. Consumer protection. 5. Trust. I. Title.

RA395.A3S495 2005

362.1—dc22

2004060659

The paper used in this publication meets the minimum requirements of American National Standard for Information Sciences—Permanence of Paper for Printed Library Materials, ANSI Z39.48-1984. ♾ ™

Acquisitions manager: Janet Davis; Project manager: Melissa A. Rompesky; Layout editor: Amanda J. Karvelaitis; Cover design: Betsy Pérez

Health Administration Press
A division of the Foundation of the
American College of Healthcare Executives
1 North Franklin Street, Suite 1700
Chicago, IL 60606-4425
(312) 424-2800

To my parents, Ruth and Milton Shore,
with admiration and love.

To my wife, Charlotte, who has always given me
the freedom and support to pursue my work
and the love to make it possible.
My love and appreciation cannot be returned
in any tangible ways.

To my children, Doug and Alyssa,
with pride and love that will extend forever.

Contents

Acknowledgments

THIS BOOK IS based largely on material presented in my one- and two-day executive education workshops and in my graduate course on building brand, reputation, and trust at Harvard University. I owe a great debt of gratitude to all of the healthcare professionals and students who have participated in these programs and in the process have taught me and helped me to refine my thinking.

This book could not have been written without the guidance and assistance of many people. First and foremost is my associate and collaborator of more than a decade, Holly Zellweger. A heartfelt thanks for the support and guidance that she has provided over the years, both in so many ways that can be counted and in countless ways that often cannot be counted, yet count most. I could not ask for a smarter, more talented, nor more gracious professional partner.

I also thank my senior research assistant, Rachel Anderson, an outstanding human being who has emerged as an invaluable asset to the team. Never once did she let me down; rather, she consistently went above and beyond the call of duty and in the process exceeded my expectations. She earned my trust and in the process my eternal gratitude. Also many thanks to Colleen Carroll and Cathy

Handy, both outstanding young professionals who deserve to have promising careers and rewarding lives ahead of them.

To the staff of the Center for Continuing Professional Education at the Harvard School of Public Health who worked tirelessly to both launch and sustain our Trust Initiative, I thank each and every one of you and extend a special thank you to the members of Team Trust.

My thanks to John Case, a consummate professional and a joy with whom to collaborate.

I also want to extend a special thank you to Barry Bloom and Jim Ware, dean and dean of academic affairs, respectively, at the Harvard School of Public Health. They supported me and my Center as we embarked on the school's Trust Initiative. Beyond simply supporting the Trust Initiative, they have enriched it. I thank them for placing their trust in me.

Finally, a special thanks to Janet Davis and her colleagues at Health Administration Press who have truly been a pleasure to collaborate with.

Introduction

You are a surgery patient. You have been stripped naked, stuck with needles, and hooked up to unfamiliar and often frightening machines. The people in charge are strangers, wear strange costumes—masks sometimes cover their faces—and have strange customs. They use words you do not understand. Yet they are about to knock you unconscious and cut open your body. How important is it that you trust the hospital and the people who work there?

You are a physician in a medical center. You do good work, but you cannot do it alone. Patients must follow your advice. The tests you order must be carried out properly. Pharmacists must fill your prescriptions correctly (and, yes, catch the occasional error). The operating rooms must be sterilized, the echocardiogram equipment must be in working order, and the people who send out the bills must do their job right so that you can get fully reimbursed for what you do. How important is it that you trust all of these people?

You run a managed care organization, a pharmaceutical company, a hospital service. You are a chief executive officer, a chief financial officer, a department head. Your business—healthcare—is probably the most complex enterprise on the face of the earth. The people you are responsible for deal every day with wellness and illness, life and death. Errors can (and do) lead to fatalities or permanent injuries. How important is it that all of the stakeholders who come into contact with your organization can trust it? How important is it that you trust all of the people your organization depends on to do its job? How important is it that they trust *you*?

I have been asking patients, staff, physicians, and healthcare leaders in the United States—indeed, all over the world—questions like these for some years now, and what I have learned could fill a book, it is here in the book you are holding. People who work in healthcare know in their mind and heart that trust is an essential element of their enterprise. All too often, unfortunately, they know that they and their organization are not trusted as much as they might be. They understand what it would mean to enjoy, and to leverage, a trusted reputation, but they are not sure how to go about building and maintaining one.

The Trust Initiative at Harvard University's School of Public Health, which I spearheaded, attracted executives and professionals from every sector of healthcare to its conferences and seminars. Here, too, we heard the same questions and the same desires. Healthcare leaders asked us again and again why they were not trusted anymore. They asked us, "How can we become more trustworthy?" and "How can our organization become *known* as the one that is trusted?" We compiled the information we gathered from these conferences and seminars into a book entitled *The Trust Crisis in Healthcare*, and our expectation is that more and more people will now be asking these questions. For as we will see in the chapters that follow, the trust crisis is real. We in healthcare are living in the midst of a substantial downturn in trust—you might even call it a "trust famine"—and so far we have not known what to do about it.

But there *are* solutions. Indeed, as real as the crisis is, so too is the opportunity. Healthcare professionals and organizations can learn to build trust. They can create a reputation that is based on trust. They can stand apart from their competitors because they, and only they, have unlocked the secret of the trust solution. Whereas the essays collected in *The Trust Crisis in Healthcare* describe and analyze the problem, this book offers answers. It will help you build your "trust capacity" with questions, ideas, models, and examples, and it will spell out the return on investment (ROI) that you can expect. It will show you how to eliminate trustbusters—those gremlins that undermine confidence—and implement trust builders. It will give you the strategies, tools, and techniques you need if you want to remake your department, service, or organization into the one with the reputation that people *really* know and trust.

WHY TRUST?

The first chapter of this book goes into detail about what I mean by trust and explores the many reasons why trust has always been important and why it is particularly important to healthcare right now. But first, consider just a little of what an organization and those who lead it stand to gain by building trust.

Trust Is a Mission Driver

The data are clear: trust improves medical outcomes. It is the number one predictor of loyalty to a physician's practice. Patients who trust their doctors are more likely to follow treatment protocols and are more likely to succeed in their efforts to change behavior (such as giving up smoking). As a plainspoken senior citizen in Birmingham, Alabama, put it to me, "If you don't trust your doctor, you just ain't gonna get well." But trust matters not only in the patient-doctor relationship but also in the patient–healthcare organization relationship. If the organization's patients and customers do not trust it, why would they avail themselves of its products and services? Alternatively, if they do trust it, why would they look anywhere else? The trusted organization is the one that people turn to when they are in need. In healthcare, almost by definition, the customers are people who are in need.[1]

Trust Is a Margin Driver

It is as true in healthcare as it is in any business: trusted organizations attract and keep customers. They enjoy a rapid utilization cycle; everything goes much more smoothly and efficiently in an environment in which everyone assumes all parties are trustworthy. Organizations that embody trust experience less bureaucracy, paperwork, and transaction costs because fewer reasons exist for generating them. Trusted organizations attract the best professionals, managers, and employees; they appeal to the best business partners and referring physicians. They can raise capital (whether investment or donations) more easily than their competitors. They are even forgiven their mistakes. Johnson & Johnson—one of the most trusted names anywhere in the world—experienced problems in a Puerto Rican manufacturing plant, and the government announced an investigation. Johnson & Johnson's stock dropped suddenly at the announcement, but the next day it was nearly back up to where it had been (Marcial 2002). Investors almost seemed to be saying to themselves, "Wait, this is Johnson & Johnson. We can trust this company to do the right thing." As we will see, the ROI in trust is substantial.

Mission and margin, of course, are the twin goals of any healthcare organization, and a strategy of building trustworthiness and a trusted reputation necessarily involves people from both the clinical and administrative spheres. It brings everyone together around a common purpose—no small feat in a world where clinicians and administrators too often regard one another with antagonism. But there are two other reasons why healthcare leaders ought to consider trust. One is strategic, the other quite personal.

On a strategic level, trust sets your organization apart. It is hardly news that healthcare has been changing rapidly. The traditional doctor's office has given way to the large group practice and the big hospital and medical center. Managed care has mostly replaced traditional insurance. Complex and costly new treatments and procedures have become more and more available every year. Consumers and patients find it all completely bewildering. These are all factors in the trust crisis; the data are compelling, and we explore some of the relevant research in the early chapters of this book. Marcus Welby, M.D., is long gone, and today consumers no longer know whom they can trust.

In this environment, the organization that *is* trusted stands utterly apart from the pack. Build a reputation based on trust, and you not only give the market what it so desperately wants and needs but you also establish a unique and sustainable value proposition for your organization. You will be head and shoulders above the competition. This book tells you how to get there; it shows you how to build a reputation for trust just as a company such as Volvo has built a reputation for safety. As Volvo owns the "safe car niche," the organization that owns the trust niche will own its marketplace.

On a personal level—as a unit head, medical director, or chief executive officer—what better legacy can you imagine than helping to create an organization that is trusted? There is something special about trust. It is not the latest management fad. It is not something that people value today but may not value tomorrow; on the contrary, it is an evergreen concern, one that will be as relevant in 20 years as it is at this moment. Trust is also the gold standard of an organization. Patients, employees, board members, suppliers, referring physicians, third-party payers, and everybody else who comes into contact with a trusted organization feel good about being associated with it. That feeling may be intangible, but it is priceless. The leaders who build an organization that is trusted can know that they have made a contribution not just to healthcare but to a better society. Here, too, this book shows you how. Trust is at once good medicine, good business, and exquisite leadership.

There is a crisis in healthcare, no doubt—a trust crisis. But crises present opportunities to those who can respond. Imagine for a moment what it would be like if you saw yourself not only as a clinician or business leader but also as a trust leader, and if your organization saw itself not only in the healthcare business but also in the trust business. Imagine that yours was the one organization that consumers immediately trusted, with their heads as well as their hearts, and that your trustworthiness was what distinguished you from the crowd. Imagine that you owned a reputation and a brand that people instantly associated with trust—and felt that they *could* trust.

Now, imagine proceeding from imagination to reality. How to build and maintain just such a reputation is the subject of this book.

PLAN OF THE BOOK

In a work of fiction, the author does not want to give away the ending. Because this is a nonfiction book, I want to give away not only the ending but the whole itinerary so that you will know where you are headed.

Part I examines the dimensions of the crisis. Chapter 1 describes what trust is, why it matters, and where it is lacking. Chapters 2 and 3 detail the current state of healthcare organizations and individual providers; Chapter 4 shows how the media exacerbate the situation; and Chapter 5 examines how people and institutions respond when trust erodes. When trust is under attack and an industry does not itself take the initiative to restore it, you can be sure that somebody else will step in. That is precisely what has happened. Everyone in healthcare today must operate in an environment where people regard each other with suspicion and where exposés and threats of stricter regulation are frequent.

Part II of the book is about building (or rebuilding) trust and a trusted reputation. It focuses on what organizations and those who lead them can do to respond to the crisis. What these chapters offer is not so much a 12-step program—I'm not sure there is one for this problem—as a way of thinking, combined with some practical advice about how and where to get started. Organizations need to understand what it means to position themselves around trust in the marketplace. They need to understand the connection between building capacity for trustworthy actions and building a reputation—a brand—known for trust. They need to understand how to communicate that reputation, and how to maintain it, year in and year out. The chapters in this section of the book deal with all of these topics.

So let us begin this journey. It offers the possibility of utterly transforming your practice, your service, your department, and your organization—and making it into a market leader.

NOTE

1. As this is the second time I have used the "c" word—customers—let me offer a blanket apology to the clinicians reading this book. I know that for many of you, every time a patient is referred to as a "customer," an angel dies.

REFERENCE

Marcial, G. G. 2002. "No More Tears at J&J." *Business Week* Aug. 5, 3794: 117.

PART I

The Missing Element in Healthcare

CHAPTER ONE

What Is Trust, and Why Does It Matter?

One day, you notice a leaky pipe in your basement. You are new to the city, so you get out the Yellow Pages and look up "plumbers." You call one of the numbers listed and talk to the owner, who promises to arrive later in the morning. Soon, indeed, a man you have never seen before shows up at your door. You notice that he is dressed like a plumber and carries a plumber's toolbox. Out in the driveway is a truck marked "Doug's Plumbing." So you decide to trust this complete stranger: you let him in the house and show him the basement. You believe he is probably competent to fix the leaky pipe.

But in fact, as any homeowner would tell you, your trust issues are just beginning. Will he fix the pipe permanently, or will it start to leak again as soon as he drives away? Will he charge you fairly? (And what is "fairly," anyway? You don't really know how much plumbers get these days.) Suppose he finds something else that he says needs to be repaired or replaced. Does it really need what he says, or is he just trying to get you to spend more money? Would another plumber do what he is doing and recommend what he is recommending? Perhaps he declares that he needs to go away and get some parts and come back in the afternoon, when you have to be out. Do you give him a key to your home? If your teenage daughter is going to be home, do you trust him alone in the house with her?

TRUST IS THE currency of all commerce. Its importance is obvious when we let a total stranger into our home, but in fact it permeates every transaction we make. We trust that the bank teller to whom we give $200 for deposit will not simply pocket the cash. We trust that the food the supermarket sells us is safe to eat. Francis

Fukuyama's (1996) book *Trust: The Social Virtues and the Creation of Prosperity* describes in elaborate detail how societies have prospered or failed to prosper depending on the breadth and depth of the trust bonds among people. The more trust that exists, the easier it is for everyone to do business and the greater is a country's prosperity.

But what is trust exactly? Supreme Court Justice Potter Stewart remarked that he did not need a formal judicial definition of pornography because "I know it when I see it." Most of us also know trust when we see it. We talk easily about somebody being trustworthy or untrustworthy. When asked how we can tell, we resort to folk sayings like, "You can see it in his eyes," "She just seems like somebody you can trust," or "I feel it in my heart." The ability to trust, and to assess other people's trustworthiness, probably developed early in human history as a survival skill.

Fukuyama (1996) writes that trust is "the expectation that arises within a community of regular, honest, and cooperative behavior, based on commonly shared norms, on the part of other members of that community." My own definition is slightly different: trust is an unwritten agreement between two or more parties for one party to perform a set of agreed-on activities and for the other party to perform a set of agreed-on activities *without fear of change from either party*. In other words, you believe that I will do what I said I would, and I believe the same about you. But formal definitions hardly do justice to a concept this rich. Trust is a term of art, with multiple dimensions. Understanding it requires holding it up to the light for examination.

THE TRUST FORMULA

One part of trust is obviously reliance on another person's *competence*. Returning to Doug the plumber, unless you believed that the man at your door was really capable of fixing your pipe, none of the other issues would even arise; you would not let him in your house in the first place. If he showed up dressed in a business suit and carrying a briefcase, you might have serious doubts about his competence. People's commitments are credible only if they are capable of doing what they say they will do. They must have the training, skills, experience, equipment, and whatever else may be necessary to carry out their intentions.

Even if he is capable, though, will he do a good job and charge you a reasonable price? Will he give you honest advice? Can you trust him alone in your home? All of these questions depend not on the plumber's competence but on his *conscience*. To trust other people fully, we must believe in their good intentions, their benevolence toward us. Conscience is the more important element of trust, if only because we can ordinarily take competence for granted. Most plumbers can fix a leaky pipe. Most bank tellers know how to record a deposit. The more important questions revolve around good intentions and benevolence. Will people act with our best interests at heart, or their own? Will they conceal something, or try to cheat us? If trust were to be described in a formula, it would have to be two parts conscience and one part competence:

$$\text{TRUST} = 2 \times \text{conscience} + \text{competence}$$

Still, the formula alone is only a starting point. The English poet and novelist D. H. Lawrence (1929) wrote the following in his poem "The Third Thing":

Water is H_2O
Hydrogen two parts
Oxygen one
But there is also a third thing
That makes it water.
And nobody knows what that is.

Trust, too, has other components, but we do not have to be quite so indeterminate about what they are.

Reducing Fear

Did you ever see the advertisement picturing a child walking up to a huge rhinoceros and patting it on the horn? "Trust is not being afraid even when you're vulnerable," reads the text. Make no mistake: Madison Avenue generally gets these things right. If you want to find symbols of trust, look first to children and animals. Vulnerability is nearly always an element in a situation of trust or distrust. The child may be gored by the rhinoceros. You may be gored, in a different sense, by the plumber when he tells you that you need a whole new water heater that will cost $10,000. You do not know enough to make an independent judgment, so you are vulnerable.

Minimizing Risk

If I trust you, I reduce my uncertainty about the future. Think for a moment about the remarkable way we handle the funds we set aside to live on in retirement. These funds are critically important to our lives and well-being. Yet we give them over to a bank or investment house and literally never see them; they are just numbers on a statement. And somehow we have complete confidence that the money is safer there than it would be under our mattress. We minimize our risk by placing our money with an institution recognized as having expertise in safeguarding funds; we believe we can trust the financial institution.

Knowing and Feeling Trust

Trust is both cerebral and emotive, involving both head and heart, both left brain and right brain. We say we "know" we can trust someone and also that we "feel" we can trust someone. A "bad feeling" about another person can be an indication of mistrust. Consider another example from Madison Avenue: think of the classic Allstate ad with the picture of a tiny home cupped in a pair of giant hands; "You're in good hands with Allstate." The image is designed to make us feel protected and safe, as we once were protected and made safe by our parents. It appeals to deep levels of emotion as well as to rational calculation.

Building Trust Through Intimacy

Trust is most easily built on a foundation of intimate face-to-face relationships, repeated over time. When our ancestors lived in hunting and gathering bands, they quickly learned which among their fellows they could trust to hunt game or pick berries successfully and then share the proceeds equitably with the group. When they lived in small communities and villages, they quickly learned who was competent and likely to deal fairly—and who, by contrast, was inclined to ineptitude or cheating. In both cases, people who betrayed a community's trust were likely to be dealt with harshly.

Trust in Today's World

Trust today, of course, is a different matter. We may still be able to make gut-level judgments about family, friends, coworkers, and neighborhood shopkeepers—the people whom we encounter in person every day. But that is nowhere near enough to sustain a modern society. We also must trust that the government will work effectively and in our best interests. We must trust that we can walk down the street in safety and that some other family will not set up housekeeping in our home when we are away on vacation. Trust infuses every successful society in a million different ways; without it, our fundamental institutions simply would not work.

The rub is that, in most cases, we can no longer make those judgments on the basis of face-to-face interaction. We have lost the intimate social environment that enabled us to do so in the past. Today we must trust in abstractions and institutions, in processes and procedures. We rely on surrogates and proxies. We react to politicians on the television screen as if they were in our living room. We make judgments about the trustworthiness of people we read about even though we do not know them. In the commercial world, as this book makes clear, we rely more than anything else on brands. We buy the names we know, because we trust them, thereby minimizing our risk. "A trusted brand is a continuous promise of future satisfaction," said I. O. Hockaday, Jr., former CEO of Hallmark. The notion of a *trusted brand* is something we will return to again and again in the book.

HEALTHCARE: APPLYING THE DEFINITIONS

Nowhere else in the modern world does trust matter more than in healthcare. Let us take what we have learned about trust, then, and apply it to the healthcare industry.

Competence

Maybe you can make an educated guess about your plumber's competence. After all, you can see the pipe or the water heater. But how many of us are confident making judgments about a physician's skill? Most of the time we do not even try; instead we use proxies, substitute attributes that we *can* evaluate. Did he go to a good medical school? Is she board certified? Does he take time to talk to us, and is his manner pleasant? There are two problems with reliance on such simple proxies. For one, the proxies can be misleading. A good education received 30 years ago or a pleasant manner in the office is no guarantee of competence in diagnosing and treating medical conditions. The more complex or unusual your ailment, moreover, the more questionable may be the doctor's competence. Has she ever even seen anything like this before? Has he treated this condition successfully? The other problem is the very high stakes involved. If your plumber makes a serious error, you can wind up with a wet basement. If your doctor makes a serious error, you can wind up disabled or dead. It would be nice to be sure—rather than simply hope—that the physician and the care team know exactly what they are doing.

The need for trust in technical competence is not limited to the patient-doctor relationship; it runs throughout healthcare. A hospital administrator depends on the competence of his staff. A surgeon depends mightily on the competence of her nurses and support personnel, right through to the people who clean the operating room. Everyone who works with a third-party payer depends on accurate and timely claims processing. Here, too, the more complex the situation, the greater is the reliance on trust. That hospital administrator can tell firsthand whether the food is good and the hallways are clean. He is unlikely to know how to conduct or interpret a computed tomography scan, so where radiology is concerned, the hospital is completely dependent for its success on those who can.

Conscience

Just as with the plumber, however, issues of competence are usually overshadowed by issues of conscience. "We trust a doctor not to do us deliberate injury," writes Fukuyama (1996), "because we expect him or her to live by the Hippocratic oath and the standards of the medical profession." In other words, we hold an implicit trust in the physician's benevolence. But how far does this extend? We must trust him to not only care for us properly but also to not order unnecessary tests in hopes of padding his own wallet or that of his employer. We must trust that he is paying attention, that he is not missing something purely from carelessness.

The need for trust in conscience also permeates the healthcare system, and a lack of this element of trust invariably makes itself felt. Take the issue of malpractice. The research is clear: patients sue doctors and hospitals not so much for making a mistake—in the end, everybody makes mistakes, and people realize that—but for not being straight with them, for covering up, for refusing to acknowledge the error and apologize for it. It is the breach of conscience that they are furious about, and that leads them to seek redress in court.

So it is with every element of trust. Take vulnerability. People who deal with the healthcare system are by definition vulnerable: they are always concerned about their health and well-being, they are often sick or injured, and they rarely know as much about their condition as do the professionals they are seeing. Trust reduces the fear that otherwise accompanies vulnerability. Similarly, consumers or patients are mightily concerned with minimizing risk, because those risks (illness, infection, bankruptcy, death) are otherwise so high. They want to know that they are covered by insurance. They want to know that the pills they are ingesting will actually help them, that the surgeon to whom they are entrusting their bodies has done the same procedure a thousand times before, and that the nursing home to which they send their mother will be a pleasant and safe place to live. Trust in such situations often carries the adjective "sacred"; it truly is a sacred trust that healthcare organizations assume when they provide their products and services to vulnerable patients or consumers.

Patients make judgments about trustworthiness with both head and heart. They use the same trust cues to assess the physician as they do with anybody else. Does the doctor look you in the eye? Does he seem rushed or distracted or abrupt? So it is with receptionists, nurses, and blood or X-ray technicians as well as with the representatives of managed care whom patients must talk to on the telephone. With institutions, too, patients make judgments about trust based on how they feel about a place in addition to what they know. If the nursing home smells of urine, placing a loved one to live there is out of the question. If the hospital's parking lot is full, the bathrooms dirty, and the cafeteria crowded, it may be out also, even if it is supposed to have a top-quality medical staff. Where trust is concerned, the brain is important, but if the gut does not go along, there is no trust.

Figure 1.1. The Trustbuster of Anonymity

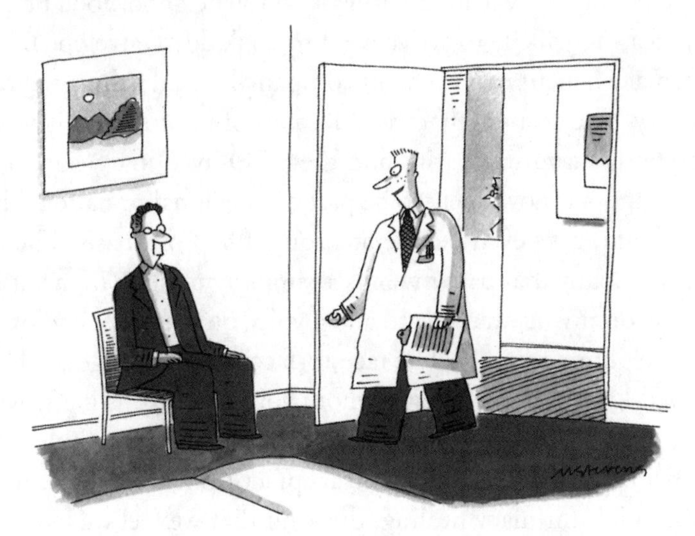

"Hi! My name is Kevin, and I'll be your doctor today."

Source: © The New Yorker Collection 1994 Mick Stevens from cartoonbank.com. All Rights Reserved.

Traditionally, healthcare was the most intimate of relationships, and hence one of the most trusting. People knew their family doctor for years and could learn whether to trust him on that face-to-face basis. "A doctor (unlike a politician or an actor) is judged only by his patients and immediate colleagues," writes the Czech author Milan Kundera (1984), "that is, behind closed doors, man to man." Adding all of the other gender combinations needed to bring Kundera's observation up to date (woman to woman, etc.), this is a fair rendition of a basic facet of patient trust. Today, the intimacy of the relationship has been compromised, and trust along with it. The patient may be ushered in, seen quickly by the doctor, then ushered out. Typically, the whole encounter takes seven minutes or less. Even the physician you see may not be "your" doctor; he or she may be your doctor's partner in a group practice or one of the many specialists to whom internists frequently refer patients (Figure 1.1).

So it is throughout healthcare. The prescription that was once prepared for me by Milt the druggist at the neighborhood pharmacy is increasingly likely to arrive in a brown padded envelope from my pharmacy benefit management company located halfway across the country. The hospital that was once part of my community—it was everybody's favorite charity, and the CEO lived in a neighborhood near mine—is now likely to be part of a regional or national health system and may even be operated on a for-profit basis. The insurance company that pays my bills is similarly remote; to me, it is just a name on my insurance card and a voice on the other end of a toll-free telephone number. The face-to-face intimacy is gone. There is no well-known human being whom you can trust. Is it any wonder that, in some parts of the country, alternative and complementary medicine has begun to catch on? Its practitioners specialize in high-touch, high-intimacy healing, the kind that we feel we have lost.

PRINCIPALS AND AGENTS

There is one more critical element of healthcare that affects trust and that makes trust even more essential in this sphere than in most others. Many interactions in the healthcare sector involve what economists call *agency relationships*, or *principal-agent relationships*. An agent is someone whose objectives are—or are supposed to be—the same as those of the principal. If I own a business and you manage it for me, you are my agent. If I am a patient and you are my doctor, you are my agent. Physicians and other caregivers are supposed to work with their patients' best interests at heart; if I am to trust you, Doctor, I must believe that this is exactly what you are doing.

But agency relationships in healthcare are always complicated and often compromised. For example, the hospital that employs a physician or the managed care company that contracts with her also expects that she will work in *their* best interests. The physician's spouse expects that he will work in the family's best interests (for example, by earning a good living and by not taking calls during the dinner hour). The incentives for agents are not always perfectly aligned with the interests of the patient. In the days of fee-for-service medicine, doctors were often accused of ordering more tests than necessary, thereby earning some extra income. In these days of managed care, they are often accused of ordering fewer than necessary, thereby saving their employer some money. In effect, service providers play multiple roles: they can induce purchases on the one hand, and they can act as a gatekeeper on the other hand, denying care or drugs that may be indicated. Ground-level clinical mistrust arises when patients feel that doctors are not acting primarily as their agents.

WHAT IS PATIENT TRUST?

This brings us to a definition of patient trust. *Patient trust* is trust in the clinical skills and knowledge of the physicians, the other professionals, and the service organizations with whom the patient comes into contact. It is confidence in the integrity of all these clinicians and organizations. And it is confidence that, whatever else they may do, they will fulfill their role as the patient's agent. The patient-physician relationship, as the *Journal of the American Medical Association* policy perspective declared a few years ago, is a "moral enterprise grounded in a covenant of trust" (Crawshaw et al. 1995). The key here, however, is that patients are dependent on trust, which is why it matters so very much.

Think of the "ABCs of patient trust" this way: in a relationship between patient and clinician, trust involves three interrelated variables. Patient A trusts clinician B to deliver valued objective C, namely high-quality, appropriate care. Clinician B is given discretion over what is done regarding clinical intervention C. Patient A and clinician B have unequal power and authority in this situation because they have unequal knowledge and expertise. A gives B even more power by bestowing some degree of trust on B; by the same token, A assumes some degree of risk by giving B discretion over

C. Because of inequity in the power relationship, a higher degree of trust is required than in relationships between equal parties.

Of course, healthcare is never so simple as just three variables. You could add in the third-party payer (D), the hospital or clinic (E), the employer that pays for the insurance (F), the pharmacy benefit management company (G), and so on, until you wound up with a veritable alphabet soup. But the point is the same: a high degree of trust is necessary precisely because what we are talking about here is healthcare. And a high degree of trust is desired by the people—the patients—whom healthcare is designed to serve.

THE ROI OF TRUST: WHY TRUST MATTERS TO ORGANIZATIONS

I remarked in the Introduction that trust is both a mission driver and a margin driver. The healthcare organization that leads its market and that operates effectively and efficiently will be a successful organization. It will also successfully pursue its mission and generate the margin it needs to operate in a competitive marketplace. One way of analyzing why trust matters to an organization's success is to calculate its return on investment (ROI). The ROI may be difficult to quantify in the case of an intangible asset such as trust, but there is no doubt that it is large. Even the most skeptical of chief financial officers can be convinced of the importance of a focus on trust.

If we go back to the essential experience of healthcare, we find that consumers—patients—must subject themselves to intimate, sometimes frightening, procedures and must follow advice that they are unlikely to understand. The products and services that constitute healthcare—doctors' exams, tests, pharmaceuticals, surgical procedures—are typically produced or performed in large, impersonal, institutional settings. A cacophony of voices in the marketplace is urging the consumer to take this or that pill, utilize this or that hospital, sign up for this or that insurance plan. Even physicians have begun to advertise.

Figure 1.2. Trust Brand Dependency Model

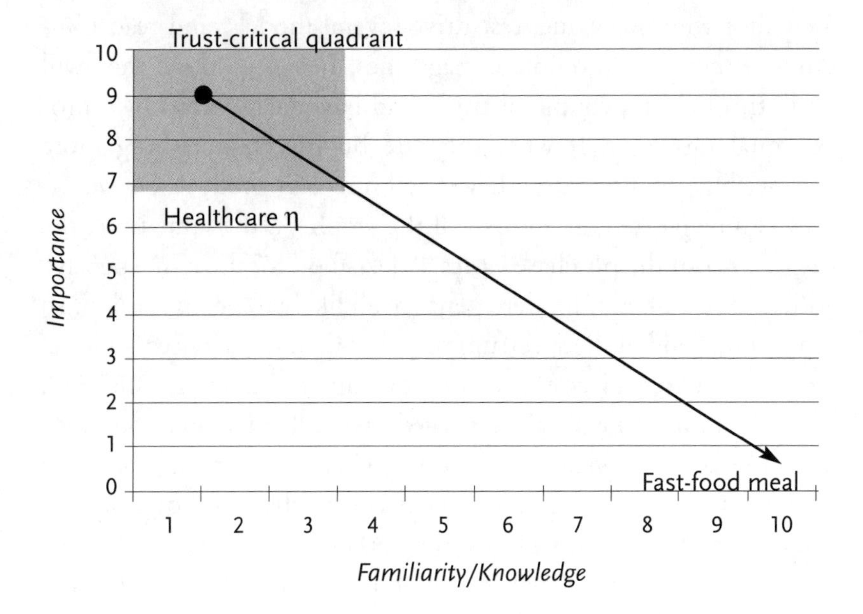

Source: © 2005, David A. Shore.

Suppose your organization stood out in this bewildering marketplace as the one that consumers knew they could trust. Across all industries, 56 percent of consumers say they will decide to purchase something simply because it was made by a company they trust (Macrae and Uncles 1997). In one recent major proprietary industry study by a large consumer healthcare company, a whopping 94 percent of consumers and 95 percent of healthcare professionals said that trust is "extremely" or "very" important. If you run a trusted organization, you will attract and keep your customers, which, after all, is the first job of any organization. Just as trust is the top predictor of loyalty to a physician's practice, it is also likely to be the top predictor of loyalty to any organization in the business of healthcare.

Another way of understanding the power of trust in the marketplace is to consider the concept of *brand dependency* (Figure 1.2).

When faced with any choice, consumers have more or less knowledge about what they are buying. If it is a car, they may talk to a neighbor who owns one, test-drive several models, and read *Consumer Reports* or automobile magazines. If it is a house, they will walk through it a couple of times and have it inspected by a professional inspector. If what they are buying is something more arcane, like legal services, they may know less about it. So *knowledge* can be plotted on one axis of the graph. At the same time, the *importance* of the purchase varies. A fast-food meal, an inexpensive gift, or a box of laundry detergent are all likely to be on the "not so important" end of the spectrum. Legal or financial services, a home, and an expensive piece of jewelry are all up on the "important" end. Healthcare, as you will have surmised, is usually high on importance and low on knowledge—precisely where consumers are most dependent on a trusted brand. That is why the healthcare organization that owns trust will own its market.

But trust has beneficial effects on an organization that go well beyond even this powerful attraction. Among them are the following:

- *Trust allows the organization to establish itself as an employer of choice*—to attract the best clinicians, managers, and employees. Look at the Great Place to Work corporate survey that appears in *Fortune* magazine every year, which gets a great deal of attention in the business world. Trust is a dominant variable and is one of the most heavily weighted. In fact, the Great Place to Work survey is, at its foundation, a Trust Index. According to the methodology, an organization simply cannot be a great place to work if it does not score well in three trust categories: credibility, respect, and fairness.
- *Trust gives an organization easier access to capital.* The scandals and investigations that plagued for-profit healthcare organizations in 2002, 2003, and 2004 scared away investors and caused many companies' stock prices to plummet. Similar troubles in not-for-profit organizations have scared away

donors and grant-making organizations. The trusted healthcare institution, whether for-profit or not-for-profit, is one that people want to invest in or support.

- *Trust appeals to key stakeholders.* Because healthcare is such a complex business, all organizations have additional key stakeholders other than customers and employees. For a hospital, one key stakeholder group is referring physicians. For a managed care organization, key stakeholders include both employers (who buy the product) and providers (who deliver the service). Trusted organizations find it easier to partner with these stakeholders.
- *Trust affects the attitude of regulators.* Healthcare is one of the most heavily regulated industries anywhere; it is subject to a bevy of federal, state, and local rules. Regulators always have a choice as to where to put their resources: they can be aggressive in their enforcement, or they can put their faith in the good word of a given organization. When an organization enjoys a reputation for trust, which is more likely?
- *Trust allows people in organizations to work together effectively.* In healthcare, many different kinds of people are asked to collaborate in a difficult and demanding enterprise. The prickly relationships that often characterize the business—nurses versus physicians, managed care organizations versus pharmaceutical companies, patients versus insurance companies, administrators versus clinicians—reflect an absence of trust. How much easier would it be for everyone if they knew that their organization, at least, could be trusted?
- *Trust reduces what economists call transaction costs.* Rules and regulations, due diligence, forms, and verifications all create extra costs for everybody, and many of them exist because not everybody can be trusted. No single organization can eliminate these transaction costs, but every organization can reduce them by building an internal culture of trust.
- *Trust offers organizations a protective moat* as well as a competitive moat. When errors occur—and they always do—a trusted

organization is more likely to be given the benefit of the doubt. Remember the anecdote about Johnson & Johnson and its Puerto Rican manufacturing facility mentioned in the Introduction.

- *Trust allows organizations to pursue rapid-cycle improvement.* Every organization in healthcare these days, without exception, is faced with the challenge of reducing errors and improving quality. The most effective method is to engineer a series of experiments aimed at producing positive change—the so-called Plan-Do-Study-Act cycle (Berwick and Nolan 1998). These are far easier to carry out in a trusting environment, and nearly impossible to carry out effectively in an atmosphere of distrust.
- *Finally, trust allows organizations to take on challenging projects*: a new product or service, a new wing for a hospital, research into a knotty problem or procedure, and so forth. Healthcare professionals everywhere thrive on the difficult challenge, but only if they truly believe that the organization taking it on can be trusted to see it through and to manage it effectively.

These factors should convince even the hardest-nosed financial officer that an investment in trust is an investment worth making. Trust is good business. But it is much more as well. One of the most basic human emotions—and one of the most basic human needs—is hope. A feeling of hopelessness and helplessness can plague people as they find their way through the jumble of healthcare organizations. In this context trust can stand out like a beacon, as a source of hope. As we will see in the following chapter, trust is sorely lacking—and it is desperately wanted.

REFERENCES

Berwick, D. M., and T. W. Nolan. 1998. "Physicians as Leaders in Improving Health Care: A New Series in *Annals of Internal Medicine*." *Annals of Internal Medicine* 128: 289–92.

Crawshaw, R., D. E. Rogers, E. D. Pellegrino, R. J. Bulger, G. D. Lundberg, L. R. Bristow, C. K. Cassel, and J. A. Barondess. 1995. "Patient-Physician Covenant." *Journal of the American Medical Association* 273 (19): 1153.

Fukuyama, F. 1996. *Trust: The Social Virtues and the Creation of Prosperity*, 26. New York: Free Press.

Kundera, M. 1984. *The Unbearable Lightness of Being: A Novel*, 183–84. Repr., New York: HarperCollins, 1999.

Lawrence, D. H. 1929. "The Third Thing." In *Pansies*, 26. Repr., Amsterdam, The Netherlands: Fredonia Books, 2002.

Macrae, C., and M. D. Uncles. 1997. "Rethinking Brand Management." *Journal of Product and Brand Management* 6: 64–77.

CHAPTER TWO

The Trust Crisis and Healthcare Organizations

Trust is like the air we breathe. When it's present, nobody really notices. But when it's absent everybody notices.

—*Warren Buffett*

ALCOHOLICS ANONYMOUS IS an effective organization in part because it insists that its members face reality before they do anything else. They must surrender to the notion that they have a problem, that their lives have become unmanageable, and that their problem will not go away by itself. So it is with trust. The healthcare system was trusted for so long that its leaders are loathe to admit that they have lost much of the public's trust. To recover—and they can recover—they must admit the extent of the problem and face it head-on. They must acknowledge that the problem of trust has impaired their work, that it has become an impediment to their stated objectives.

How bad is the situation? In my talks, I often use a glass for a prop and pour it half full of water. "This is the trust glass," I tell the audience, "and we are going to talk about whether it is half full or half empty." But perhaps the metaphor should be less ambiguous. The sad truth is that healthcare is in the middle of a trust famine, a continuing, long-term decline in trust, one that will not easily be reversed. The data on this topic are quite compelling.

THE TRUST FAMINE

"I am going to name some institutions in this country. As far as the people running these institutions are concerned, would you say you have a great deal of confidence, only some confidence, or hardly any confidence at all in them?" This question and similar ones have been put to Americans by polling organizations for many years, and the results give a good general indication of the extent to which Americans trust their society's central institutions. Year-to-year figures naturally fluctuate depending on what is in the news, but where healthcare is concerned, the long-term trend is quite clear. In 1966, 73 percent of Americans expressed a "great deal of confidence" in leaders of medical institutions. By 2004, that figure had dropped to less than half of the 1966 total, to 32 percent. And though the 32 percent was a modest improvement over the all-time low of 20 percent in the early 1990s, the trend line has hardly made gains (Figure 2.1). Medicine started out with higher public confidence, had a steeper decline in confidence, and by 2004 ended up 41 percent lower than the 1966 levels, compared with the other institutions polled during the polling period, which only dropped 22 percent. Confidence in medicine has without a doubt substantially eroded, and it is unlikely to improve significantly in the near future.

The erosion in trust has affected all age groups. Trust among the elderly—those 65 and over—dropped 4 percentage points from the 1970s to the 1990s, the smallest decline of any age group. Trust among the middle aged dropped considerably more; the largest decline was among people 35 to 64. When we examine the figures for 2000, which are more or less typical, we find that there is remarkably little variation among different social groups. Men express somewhat more confidence in healthcare than women do. People living in the southern United States express somewhat less confidence than people elsewhere. Those who say they are in excellent health are more trusting than those who are in poorer health. Ironically, sicker people need to trust more but actually trust less.

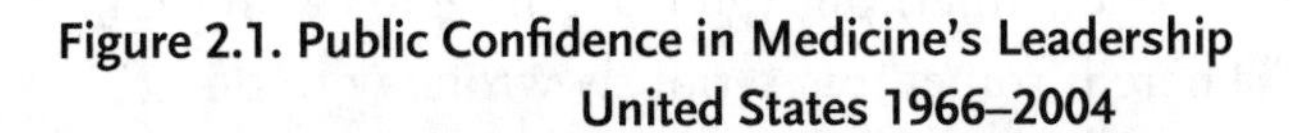

Figure 2.1. Public Confidence in Medicine's Leadership
United States 1966–2004

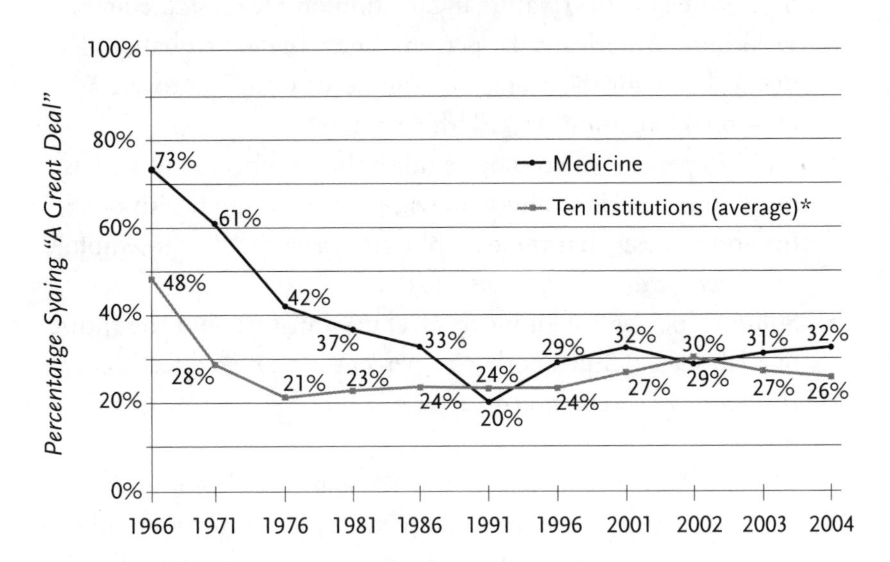

* Average of ratings for those running the following ten institutions: the military, medicine, The U.S. Supreme Court, major educational institutions such as colleges and universities, organized religion, major companies, the executive branch of the federal government, the press, Congress, and organized labor. Organized religion was not asked in 1996; organized labor was not asked in 1991 or 1996.

Source: Data from Harris, 1966–2004. Adapted and updated from Robert Blendon, presentation at "The Public's Health: A Matter of Trust Symposium," 2002, Harvard University School of Public Health.

Overall, however, the differences are relatively small. "The erosion of faith in medicine is not restricted to certain specific social sectors, such as African-Americans, the poor, or those with health problems," writes Prof. Pippa Norris (2005) of Harvard University's John F. Kennedy School of Government, "but instead has occurred fairly uniformly throughout all major groups in America."

When confidence in a whole set of institutions declines in this manner, the resulting lack of trust manifests itself in dozens of different ways. The following are some examples:

- The vast majority of Americans (79 percent) agree with the statement, "There is something seriously wrong with our healthcare system" (National Coalition on Health Care 1997).
- Even more Americans (87 percent) agree that "the quality of medical care for the average person needs to be improved" (National Coalition on Health Care 1997).
- Only 36 percent of employers think the healthcare industry is heading in the right direction with respect to the health benefits and services that these employers currently offer to employees (*Consortium Connection* 2003).
- Some 40 percent of employers feel pessimistic about the future of healthcare, while another 22 percent have mixed feelings (*Consortium Connection* 2003).

The anecdotes people read in the newspapers only reinforce these dour views. A surgeon leaves the operating room in the middle of surgery to visit his bank. A major cancer center makes a medication error and a patient dies. Pharmacists are accused of diluting medications, physicians of bilking Medicare out of billions of dollars, pharmaceutical scientists of fudging lab results. Whole health systems are racked by charges of fraud and abuse. A notable example, the HealthSouth story, is described on the following page.

Each part of the healthcare sector experiences its own particular brand of mistrust. Each part also participates in its own plummeting trust by allowing specific *trustbusters* to occur. Trustbusters are reasons why people come to distrust a particular healthcare provider or institution, and by extension all similar entities, or worse yet, the healthcare industry as a whole. We will consider the plight of organizations in this chapter, and the situation of individual providers in the next.

Managed Care

Managed care dates back to 1938, when California industrialist Henry Kaiser was employing many thousands of men to build the Grand

The HealthSouth Story

HealthSouth Corp., founded in 1984, had grown to be a company with $4 billion in revenues by the time it collapsed in early 2003. It was the largest operator of rehabilitation centers and outpatient surgery centers in the United States. It worked in partnership with high-profile physicians such as James Andrews and Larry Lemak, whose Alabama Sports Medicine and Orthopedic Center treated sports superstars. It was building a new hospital—christened the "digital hospital" for its aspiration to state-of-the-art computer technology—in its hometown of Birmingham, Alabama. At its peak, the company claimed a market value of more than $12 billion. HealthSouth's CEO, Richard Scrushy, had become not only a very rich man but also a local celebrity, donating millions of dollars to charitable causes.

The first chink in HealthSouth's apparent success story came in July 2002, when a Scrushy associate named William A. Massey, Jr., committed suicide. Massey was later alleged to have stolen as much as $500,000 from Scrushy. In August, the company announced that its profit would fall short of projections by $175 million; its stock plunged 58 percent in two days, and the Securities and Exchange Commission (SEC) launched an investigation. Six months later, in March 2003, the SEC filed a $1.4 billion fraud suit against Scrushy and others, alleging that the company had cooked its books over a period of years in order to inflate its profits. Over the next seven weeks, the Justice Department recorded guilty pleas from 11 of Scrushy's associates, including all five of the people who had served as HealthSouth's chief financial officers. As this book went to press, the investigation was continuing amid speculation that criminal charges might be filed against Scrushy. HealthSouth—under new leadership—was fighting to recover.

Interestingly, at no time did any allegations surface about the quality of the healthcare offered at HealthSouth facilities. Physicians who partnered with the company seemed content. ("We don't have plans other than business as usual with HealthSouth," said Dr. Lemak in April 2003.) No unusual number of patients were complaining about poor-quality care. But the HealthSouth saga is the most dramatic example to date of the breaches of organizational trust that can occur in America's mixed and turbulent healthcare enterprise. A for-profit

(continued on following page)

company, HealthSouth grew partly by consolidating what had been a local, small-scale business (rehabilitation centers), then using its apparently inflated stock to finance a host of acquisitions. It necessarily became dependent on Wall Street's approval to maintain the stock price, and when the earnings were not sufficient to justify the stock, the company's officers apparently decided to make them look better.

The result, of course, was a betrayal of HealthSouth's thousands of honest employees; its healthcare professionals; and its many, many patients, all of whom had no reason to believe that the company was anything but trustworthy. It was not.

Coulee Dam on the Columbia River in central Washington. Kaiser asked a physician named Sidney Garfield to create a prepaid healthcare plan for his employees. The plan would focus on preventive care, not just curing the sick and fixing up the injured. It would cover workers' families as well as the workers themselves. That plan eventually evolved into Kaiser Permanente, the large health maintenance organization (HMO). A few other plans partly modeled on Kaiser came into existence as well. One in Boston was known as Harvard Community Health Plan; it, too, grew into a good-sized HMO before metamorphosing and dividing into a large insurer (Harvard Pilgrim Health Care) and a substantial medical group practice (Harvard Vanguard Medical Associates). In 1973, the federal government passed the Health Maintenance Organization Act, requiring large employers to offer their employees the choice of an HMO as well as traditional indemnity insurance plans. After that, HMOs proliferated (Cutler 2005).

However, managed care today is not in good shape. Its troubles show up in the data, which show that HMO enrollees continue to be less trusting than people enrolled in other types of health plans (Center for Studying Health System Change 2002). Only 13 percent of poll respondents say they have a "great deal" or "quite a lot" of confidence in HMOs, down from 17 percent in 1999 (Robinson and Blizzard 2002). Nearly half (about 46 percent) believe that the trend toward managed care is a bad thing (HFM 2001). Even more believe that the trend will negatively affect the quality of medical care. HMOs' troubles also show up in the popular culture. Managed care executives typically rank just above tobacco company executives in questions about which occupations people trust and respect. Television shows and movies such as *John Q* regularly portray managed care executives as villains. (We will explore this phenomenon in greater depth in Chapter 4.) Managed care is the butt of frequent jokes. A *New Yorker* cartoon from a few years back shows children at camp gathered around the campfire; one has just finished telling a story. "Very scary, Jennifer," says the counselor. "Does anyone else have an HMO horror story?" (See box, "In the Beginning," page 28).

Asking what consumers object to about managed care is not quite the right question; a better one is what consumers do not object to. One major trustbuster derives from the principal-agent relationship we discussed in the previous chapter. When a physician is employed by a managed care organization, patients perceive the doctor as less than independent. They worry about whether he or she has the patient's—and only the patient's—best interests at heart. Interestingly, Dr. Dana Safran and her colleagues have found that the structure of a managed care organization matters a great deal in this regard. Staff-model HMOs—those that employ physicians on staff—engender the greatest distrust. Other, more flexible plans, such as independent practice association/network and other "open" models, engender less distrust (Safran et al. 2000). The more restrictive the plan, in other words, the less independent the physician is perceived to be and the less trust the patient feels in the doctor. When HMOs are perceived to be controlling the practice of doctors by employing them or restricting their behavior, the principal-agent relationship is compromised. For-profit healthcare presents a particular difficulty because patients are easy to exploit, given the specialized education required to understand medical decisions and the possible incentive to deny care in favor of the bottom line. Therefore, the less restrictive a managed care plan appears to be, the more it appears to be trustworthy.

In the Beginning

In the beginning, God populated the earth with broccoli and cauliflower and spinach, green and yellow and red vegetables of all kinds, so man and woman would live long and healthy lives.

Then, using God's great gifts, Satan created Ben & Jerry's and Krispy Kreme, and Satan said, "You want chocolate with that?"

And man said, "Yeah!" And woman said, "And another one with sprinkles!" and they gained 10 pounds.

And God created healthful yogurt that woman might keep the figure that man found so fair; Satan brought forth white flour from the wheat and sugar from the cane and combined them, and woman went from size 2 to size 6.

So God said, "Try my fresh green salad." And Satan presented Thousand Island dressing and garlic toast on the side. And man and woman unfastened their belts.

God then said, "I have sent you heart-healthy vegetables and olive oil in which to cook them." And Satan brought forth deep-fried fish and chicken-fried steak so big it needed its own platter. And man gained more weight, and his cholesterol went through the roof.

God then introduced running shoes so that his children might lose extra pounds. And Satan countered with cable TV with a remote control so that man would not have to toil to change the channels. And man and woman laughed and cried before the flickering light and gained more pounds.

Then God brought forth the potato, naturally low in fat and brimming with nutrition, and Satan peeled off the healthful skin and sliced the starchy center into chips and deep-fried them, and man began to look like a blimp.

God then recommended lean beef so that man might consume fewer calories and still satisfy his appetite. And Satan created fast-food restaurants and the 99-cent double cheeseburger. Then he added, "Do you want fries with that?" and man replied "Yeah! And super size 'em." And Satan said, "It is good." And man went into cardiac arrest. God sighed and created quadruple bypass surgery.

And Satan created HMOs.

Note: This entertaining story was sent to me electronically many times by healthcare colleagues and members of managed care plans. Its author is anonymous, as far as I know.

A second trustbuster is perceived interference in the doctor-patient relationship, even when the physician is thought to be independent of the managed care organization. The patient asks the doctor what she recommends. The doctor recommends some tests or procedures but wonders whether the patient's insurance will cover them. The patient contacts the health plan and suddenly finds that he must go through a "medical necessity" review. (In my discussions with managed care executives, they acknowledge that these reviews are one of the great dissatisfiers of managed care.) If he is turned down, it is a safe bet that the doctor will throw up her hands and blame the HMO for its stinginess, thereby reinforcing the patient's belief that the HMO is interfering with the doctor's medical judgment.

A third trustbuster is the for-profit status of many managed care organizations. Even not-for-profit HMOs tend to act much like businesses, so consumers feel that these organizations are more interested in saving money, or in rewarding their investors, than they are in providing top-quality care. Many of the articles in a 1999 book, provocatively titled *Making a Killing: HMOs and the Threat to Your Health*, made precisely the case that the top priority of HMOs is not maximizing patients' health but controlling costs by limiting the use of resources (Court and Smith 1999). Ironically, the better HMOs do financially, the less consumers may trust them. This is not surprising when they see situations of managed care organizations dropping more than 2 million unprofitable Medicare patients, while earning record profits during the same time period.[1] In fact, several studies report that roughly half of the people surveyed thought that the growth of for-profit ownership of health plans and hospitals was a "bad thing" (Schlesinger, Mitchell, and Gray). And in another study, they were judged to be more untrustworthy and overpriced than non-profits. For-profit hospitals were not trusted to restrain spending on unnecessary procedures or not discharge sick patients if their insurance runs out. For-profit health plans were not trusted to charge fairly for insurance. The same study found that overall expectations of quality care were higher for for-profit organizations, and that expectations were higher for the group respondents who could not define ownership. The study authors suggest that this expectation of higher quality might be related to perceiving non-profit healthcare as charity care.[2] It could also be an expectation that a for-profit business is more efficient, modern, and effective than a non-profit organization. In any case, the profit motive is overwhelmingly associated with overcharging and untrustworthiness.

The more profitable a for-profit managed care organization is perceived to be, the less trustworthy it appears. This inverse relationship between trustworthiness and financial success does not apply to other corporate entities. Can you imagine any other corporation—GE, for instance—being villified for financial success? An unspoken industry assumption, and a public one, is that a managed care company's healthy profit margin suggests that money was taken away from patient care to amass it. With more and more for-profit healthcare corporations, this apparent conflict between patient care and financial profits is the biggest trustbuster faced by for-profit healthcare entities, especially managed care organizations.

Hospitals and Health Systems

Not so long ago, hospitals enjoyed a privileged place in American society. They were seen as clean, friendly places where the injured were healed and the sick made well. Big donors competed to endow new wings or laboratories and to sit on hospital boards as trustees. The public trusted hospitals; in polls, people expressed few concerns about the quality of care offered by them. Ironically, some of this trust may have been misplaced. Nearly 30 years ago, the social critic Ivan Illich was already arguing that hospitals make people sicker rather than better (Illich 1976). Illich offered evidence that as many as 20 percent of all patients who entered a university hospital contracted an iatrogenic (doctor-caused) illness. "Despite good intentions and claims to public service, a military officer with a similar record of performance would be relieved of his command, and a restaurant or amusement center would be closed by the police" (Illich 1976, 23).

Today, at any rate, the level of trust in hospitals has plummeted. Fully 75 percent of the public believes that hospitals (as well as insurers) are not prepared for the demands of tomorrow's consumers (O'Dell 2002). Only 40 percent of consumers trust hospitals for their healthcare information (VHA 2000). It is telling that the American Hospital Association (AHA), which periodically issues "Reality Check" qualitative studies examining "America's Message to Hospitals and Health Systems," devoted a recent report to the subject of trust. "Searching for Trust" was the title—and the message of the study was that trust was hard to find (AHA 1998–1999).

Some of the reasons for the decline—the trustbusters—reflect broad changes in healthcare. Many hospitals themselves are now run on a for-profit basis, and eight out of ten Americans believe that the quality of medical care is being compromised in the interest of profit (National Coalition on Health Care 1997). Many have become part of big national chains, never very popular with the public. But often the trustbusters reflect mediocre hospital management. The following are some examples:

- Hospital patients continue to die in large numbers from preventable errors. We will take up medical errors in more detail in the following chapter; for the moment, it is worth remembering that somewhere between 50,000 and 180,000 people die each year from iatrogenic causes. This issue has finally begun to get serious attention from researchers and organizations such as the Institute of Medicine. Ironically, the resulting publicity—though good for trust in the long run, if it encourages hospitals to improve their performance—is certainly damaging to trust in the short run.
- Hospital finances have been squeezed by managed care organizations and Medicare on the one hand and by the need to

provide unreimbursed care for the uninsured on the other. Many hospitals have responded to the squeeze by cutting costs. Some of the effects are seemingly minor but go far toward undermining trust: dirty hallways and bathrooms, overflowing garbage cans, poor food service. Other effects can be devastating. One study, for example, found that patients' risk of dying after surgery increased by 14 percent when the patient's nurse was responsible for six beds rather than four. The risk increased by more than 30 percent if the nurse covered eight beds (Aiken et al. 2002).

- Some hospitals have responded to the cost squeeze by more aggressively collecting on outstanding charges. A 2003 article in the *Wall Street Journal*, for instance, documented one (not-for-profit) hospital's attempts to collect an outstanding debt from a low-income, 77-year-old widower by filing suit against him (Lagnado 2003).

Few healthcare professionals in most hospitals seem to be worrying about such trustbusters. The AHA report "Searching for Trust" asked hospital executives, "Who is in charge of managing the reputation of your hospital or health system?" but the only answer they could come up with seemed to be, "Everyone and no one." The story with other healthcare organizations need not be told in as much detail, because the essentials are much the same.

Pharmaceutical Companies

Consumers have a love-hate relationship with pharmaceutical companies: they snap up the drugs that help cure their ailments, but they do not feel warmly about the organizations that make them. A Harris Poll regularly asks people if they think pharmaceutical companies do a good job of serving their customers. Positive responses to the question dropped 30 percent between 1997 and 2003 (Taylor 2003). "It's ironic," wrote columnist Alan Murray in 2003, "that an industry that does so much good has developed a public image that is so unrelentingly bad."

A particular sore point with consumers is the cost of medications. As Congress debated a bill in 2003 that would provide partial drug benefits to Medicare recipients, the consumer group Families USA issued a report pointing out that prices of the prescription drugs taken by most seniors rose by more than four times the previous year's inflation rate (Families USA 2003). "These kinds of numbers, I believe, are immoral," said Sen. Debbie Stabenow (D-Mich) to a reporter. "Medicine is different. It's not like buying a car or tennis shoes or peanut butter" (Lueck 2003). It is safe to say that Sen. Stabenow's opinions reflected the views of millions of Americans.

The attitude of managed care organizations toward pharmaceutical manufacturers may be even more negative than the attitudes of consumers. In a proprietary study of managed care medical directors by a major pharmaceutical company, for instance, most characterized the pharmaceutical industry as "aggressive," "greedy," "self-serving," and "not to be trusted." Few felt that they could truly trust the pharmaceutical companies to keep the best interests of patients or managed care organizations in mind. The industry's direct-to-consumer advertising has often soured its relationship with physicians as well; more and more, consumers are coming into the doctor's office, ad in hand, asking for a particular medication—and challenging the doctor's judgment if he or she will not prescribe it.

Pharmacy Benefit Management Companies

Pharmacy benefit management companies (PBMs) first appeared in the late 1980s and early 1990s; they manage drug benefits for individuals on behalf of their employer or their managed care organization. A number of large PBMs have provoked criticism for both their size and their methods of operation. One trustbuster revolves around access rebates, which are discounts on drugs offered by the manufacturer in return for listing of that drug on the PBM's formulary. A second is market share rebates. PBMs by their very size can influence a drug's market share, which in turn has an effect on its manufacturer's financial health and stock price, so the PBM gets a better price if it moves a drug's share in a positive direction. These rebates, along with a variety of other practices, mean that the PBMs are closely tied to the pharmaceutical companies. How closely? No one knows, because the terms of the rebates and the amounts of money involved have been closely guarded secrets.

The result, not surprisingly, is a deep suspicion on the part of their customers and representatives of the public. Lawsuits have accused the PBMs of violating their fiduciary duties to customers. A U.S. attorney in Philadelphia has probed what he termed "secret payments" between PBMs and pharmaceutical companies. "A growing chorus of critics says that PBMs are actually being manipulated by pricing schemes and sweetheart promotional deals to push the most expensive drugs on the market," said an article in *Managed Care* magazine, "an explosive political issue for companies at a time when Congress is anxiously hunting for ways to legislate caps on the skyrocketing cost of drugs" (Carroll 2002).

Insurance Companies

These days, of course, there is not as much distinction as there once was between traditional insurance companies such as Aetna and CIGNA and managed care organizations; most of the traditional companies offer managed care plans of their own. But the insurers do not want you to tar them with the same brush. As one executive put it to me, "While insurance companies aren't well thought of...they are one step above managed care!" Like managed care organizations, however, insurance companies are mistrusted by both patients and physicians. More than 50 percent of Americans say health insurance companies do a "bad job" of serving the needs of patients (Taylor 2003). In one large proprietary industry study, a trust-related issue turned out to be the number one concern among health insurance plan members, specifically, the perception that the insurance company interferes with the physician's decisions.

Like many players in the healthcare sector, most insurance companies are for-profit organizations. This fact cuts both ways. As mentioned, many people are dubious that a company responsible to its investors can have patients' best interests at heart. It is probably not lost on those who come across CIGNA's well-known tagline highlighting the business of caring, that the company puts "business" before "caring." Yet some of the best financial results have been turned in by companies that provide patient-centered service. UnitedHealth Group, which owns one of Wall Street's best-performing stocks, saw five years of consistently increasing profits between 1999 and 2004. Yet UnitedHealth has gone far toward limiting or removing gatekeepers on its members—a popular move with patients—and its four core values are all patient focused (UnitedHealth 2004). Wellpoint has also enjoyed a healthy stock appreciation and introduced physician incentives tied to quality of care. So doing good and doing well are not necessarily exclusive.

THE EMPTY TRUST GLASS

Despite the occasional bright spot, all of this adds up to a system that many suspect has lost its moral moorings. I use the word "system" loosely in this statement, because the United States does not really have a healthcare system. The United Kingdom has a healthcare system; so does Canada. The United States has a collection of provider organizations and payers that are fragmented and often in competition with one another. Various sectors typically view others as competitors, enemies, or (at best) necessary evils, and infrequently as allies in the delivery of service. The system may be seen as consisting of multiple dichotomies: physicians versus hospitals, providers versus payers, government (at various levels) versus providers, hospitals versus accreditation bodies, profit-seeking companies versus nonprofit organizations. The list could go on, but the point is simple: nearly all of these relationships are characterized by a low degree of trust. And the consumer—the patient—who is the ultimate beneficiary or victim of the enterprise, has the least trust of all. The trust glass of provider organizations, in short, is half empty at best. The time to refill it has come.

NOTES

1. "Medicare HMO Fiasco: Few Options Available for the Nearly One Million Seniors to be Dropped from HMOs by Year-End." Nov. 8, 2000. Weiss Ratings Inc. [Online article; retrieved 12/15/04.] http://www.weissratings.com/news/Ins_Medigap/20001108medigap.htm.
2. Schlesinger, Mitchell, and Gray.

REFERENCES

2001. "Managed Care Backlash May be Waning." *Healthcare Financial Management* 55 (9): 21.

Aiken, L. H., S. P. Clarke, D. M. Sloane, J. Sochalski, and J. H. Silber. 2002. "Hospital Nurse Staffing and Patient Mortality, Nurse Burnout, and Job Dissatisfaction." *Journal of the American Medical Association* 288 (16): 1991.

American Hospital Association. 1998–1999. "Searching for Trust: America's Message to Hospitals and Health Systems." *Reality III, National Focus Group Research.*

Carroll, J. 2002. "When Success Sours: PBMs Under Scrutiny." *Managed Care* 11 (9): 20–26. [Online article; retrieved 5/11/04.] http://www.managedcaremag.com/archives/0209/0209.pbms.html.

Center for Studying Health System Change. 2002. "Who Do You Trust? American's Perceptions of Health Care, 1997–2001." In *Tracking Report*, vol. 3, p. 1. Washington, DC: Center for Studying Health System Change.

Consortium Connection. 2003. "Understanding Market Expectations." *Consortium Connection* Winter: 6.

Court, J., and F. Smith. 1999. *Making a Killing: HMOs and the Threat to Your Health*. Monroe, ME: Common Courage Press.

Cutler, C. 2005. "The Changing Relationship Between Health Plans and Their Members." In *The Trust Crisis in Healthcare: Causes, Consequences and Cures*, edited by D. A. Shore. New York: Oxford University Press.

Families USA. 2003. "Out of Bounds: Rising Prescription Drug Prices for Seniors." [Online article; retrieved 2/24/05.] http://www.familiesusa.org/site/DocServer /Out_of_Bounds.pdf?docID=1522.

Illich, I. 1976. *Medical Nemesis: The Exploration of Health*. New York: Pantheon Books.

Lagnado, L. 2003. "Twenty Years and Still Paying—Jeanette White Is Long Dead but Her Hospital Bill Lives on; Interest Charges, Legal Fees." *Wall Street Journal* March 13, B1.

Lueck, S. 2003. "Drug Prices Far Outpace Inflation." *Wall Street Journal* July 10, D2.

Murray, A. 2003, "Drug Import Vote Is Cue for Industry to Change Its Ways." *Wall Street Journal* July 29, A4.

National Coalition on Health Care. 1997. "How Americans Perceive the Health Care System: A Report on a National Survey." Washington, DC: National Coalition on Health Care.

Norris, P. 2004. "Skeptical Patients: Performance, Social Capital, and Culture." Presented at "The Public's Health: A Matter of Trust" Symposium. Boston. Data derived from the NORC U.S. General Social Survey 1973–2000, sample pooled by decade.

O'Dell, G. 2002. "2002 American Hospital Association Environmental Assessment." *Hospitals & Health Networks* 76 (9): 61.

Robinson, J., and R. Blizzard. 2002. "Americans and Managed Care: Time For Change?" [Online article; retrieved 11/12/04.] *The Gallup Poll Tuesday Briefing*, July 16. http://www.gallup.com/poll/content/login.aspx?ci=6403.

Safran, D. G., W. H. Rogers, A. R. Tarlov, T. Inui, D. A. Taira, J. E. Montgomery, J. E. Ware, and C. P. Slavin. 2000. "Organizational and Financial Characteristics of Health Plans: Are They Related to Primary Care Performance?" *Archives of Internal Medicine* 160 (1): 69–76.

Schlesinger, M., S. Mitchell, and B. H. Gray. "Public Expectations of Nonprofit and Fot-Profit Ownership in American Medicine: Clarifications and Implications." *Health Affairs* 23 (6): 181–91.

Taylor, H. 2003. "Supermarkets, Food Companies, Hospitals, and Banks Top the List of Industries Doing Good Job for Their Customers." The Harris Poll, #31. [Online article; retrieved 2/24/05.] http://www.harrisinteractive.com/harris_poll/index.asp?pid=379.

UnitedHealth Group. 2004. "About United Health Group Mission and Values." [Online article; retrieved 2004.] http://www.unitedhealthgroup.com/about/val.htm.

VHA, Inc. 2000. "Consumer Demand for Clinical Quality: The Giant Awakens." *Research Series—Consumer Demand for Clinical Quality* 3: 16. [Online report; retrieved 11/12/04.] https://www.vha.com/research/public/consumerdemandforclinicalquality.pdf.

CHAPTER THREE

The Trust Crisis and Individual Providers

Relationships of trust depend on our willingness to look not only to our own interests, but also the interests of others.

—Peter Farquharson

IF INSPIRING TRUST is your goal, the professions of insurance salesperson and advertising executive present a challenge. Asked to evaluate the honesty and ethical standards of people in these fields, only 12 percent of poll respondents give these occupations a "high" or "very high" rating. Nor would you want to be in auto sales, an occupation that comes in at only 7 percent (Gallup News Service 2003).

By contrast, healthcare professionals have traditionally rated relatively high in the public's esteem. In a 2003 poll, medical doctors were rated as high or very high in esteem by 68 percent of the respondents. Though their ratings had been climbing since 2000, the 2003 poll gave them the highest score they have ever received in this Gallup survey. Pharmacists scored 67 percent, and nurses an impressive 83 percent. Nurses and medical doctors ranked number one and number two among all occupations, with pharmacists ranking third (after veterinarians, who tied with medical doctors for second place) (Gallup News Service 2003).[1] Indeed, nurses rank so high that one wonders why more healthcare organizations do not promote the quality and integrity of their nursing staff, in effect making nurses the stewards of their brand. But we will get to such proposals later in the book.

The paradoxical coexistence of trust and trustbusters affects the trust glass of individual providers and the entire healthcare industry. Though healthcare professionals consistently rank high, the trust placed in them by the public is in constant danger of being undermined. We will now explore three such trustbusters.

One kind of trustbuster arises from isolated (but well-publicized) acts of criminality and inhumanity on the part of the very professionals in whom we place that trust. A nurse in New Jersey admitted to killing 40 patients (Kocieniewski 2004). A pharmacist in Kansas City confessed to diluting medications for nearly a decade (Elliott 2002). A surgeon whose last name begins with "Z" carved the initial on a woman's abdomen to mark the completion of a successful operation (Steinhauer and Wong 2000). Such anecdotes mount up over time and ultimately can erode the public's faith in the people who deliver healthcare.

Another kind of trustbuster comes from the organizational pressures described in the previous chapter. Perceptions of time spent and actual time spent or time necessary may vary significantly. A trusting patient may be less likely to perceive too little time being spent on his or her care. Be that as it may, physicians who spend an average of seven minutes with their patients will eventually find that they are not trusted as much as the old family doctor who spent 20 or 30 minutes on an office visit. Furthermore, short-staffed nursing services place so much pressure on individual nurses that some may no longer have time for the caring and personal attention that build patient trust, a cornerstone of the practice of nursing.

But the most significant threat to the public's trust in individual providers comes from systemwide issues that are lurking beneath the surface, threatening to erupt at any time. The most urgent of these issues is medical errors.

MEDICAL ERRORS

On July 2, 2001, *People* magazine ran a two-page advertisement with a large pie chart entitled "Major Causes of Death in the United States." The ad also ran in five other consumer magazines with a combined circulation of 24.6 million, including *Parents*, *Family Circle*, and *Good Housekeeping*. It was sponsored by the UnitedHealth Foundation, a not-for-profit division of UnitedHealth Group. The chart in the ad had a slice for breast cancer, a slice for vehicular accidents, and a slice for AIDS. A fourth slice, larger than any of the other two combined and nearly as large as all three put together, was simply entitled, "Oops!" The text accompanying the chart was directed at individual healthcare consumers, and warned them of the dangers of medical errors. It then provided eight practical tips for consumers to help them prevent medical errors. Within the healthcare field, the ad sparked controversy about its facts and presentation. Regardless, from the perspective of impact on the public, this was a landmark ad, in that a major player in the industry—and a company widely regarded as an innovator—was publicizing the fact that medical errors are both widespread and serious. The message could hardly be lost on patients: doctors could harm them as well as help them.

According to a study by the IOM, medical errors account for somewhere between 44,000 and 98,000 deaths a year (Kohn, Corrigan, and Donaldson 2000). My Harvard colleague, Lucian Leape, one of the foremost experts in the field, estimates that 180,000 patients a year die from adverse events, including errors and medical accidents, of which he estimates about two-thirds are preventable (Brennan et al. 1991). Barbara Starfield (2000) of Stanford University has come up with an even higher number, claiming that errors and other adverse events lead to 225,000 deaths per year (see box). From this data, Starfield determined that iatrogenic illness and injuries are the third-leading cause of death in the United States, after heart disease and cancer. All such data, moreover, are for deaths

Mind-numbing Statistics

- 12,000 deaths per year from unnecessary surgery
- 7,000 deaths per year from medication errors in hospitals
- 20,000 deaths per year from other errors in hospitals
- 80,000 deaths per year from nosocomial infections (infections originating in the hospital)
- 106,000 deaths per year from nonerror adverse effects of medication

Source: Starfield (2000).

only; they do not include adverse events that lead to disability or severe discomfort.

A comparison of accidental gun deaths with deaths caused by medical error has appeared on hundreds of Internet web sites and in chain e-mails. It has been interpreted as tragic, funny, or misrepresented, and used to support a wide range of conflicting positions. The numbers are presented roughly as follows. There are about 700,000 physicians in the United States, this student pointed out, and perhaps 120,000 accidental deaths caused by physicians each year. That works out to 0.171 deaths per physician. Meanwhile, there are 80,000,000 gun owners and about 1,500 accidental gun deaths per year, for a ratio of 0.0000188 deaths per gun owner. In other words, according to this accounting, doctors are approximately 9,000 times more dangerous than gun owners (Break the Chain 2003).

Whatever the numbers may be—and whether we take a serious or a satirical approach to publicizing them—there is no doubt that they are large and that medical errors are a terrible problem. Moreover, the cat is out of the bag: errors have become a subject for widespread research, and they are a recurrent topic of stories in the media. The more the public learns about them, the better it may be for healthcare in the long run, but the worse it is for trust in the short run. People may still hold physicians and other providers in high esteem, but they are not sure that these professionals can be trusted. They make too many mistakes.

GAMING THE SYSTEM (AND OTHER ILLS)

A second issue affecting trust is "gaming the system," or manipulating the rules of the system to some advantage, and all that it implies about how healthcare operates. A policy perspective article in the *Journal of the American Medical Association* states that medicine is "a moral enterprise grounded in a covenant of trust. . . . Physicians therefore are both intellectually and morally obliged to act as advocates for the sick wherever their welfare is threatened and for their health at all times" (Crawshaw et al. 1995). Many doctors feel this obligation acutely when their patients are not covered, or only partially covered, by insurance. In one study, 39 percent of the more than 1,000 physicians polled reported manipulating reimbursement rules to obtain coverage for services that they believed were necessary (Wynia et al. 2000). Studies like this show that physicians engage in covert advocacy tactics—for example, reporting diagnoses that are more serious than they really are so that the patient will be covered. Nor is it surprising that they do so, given the rigidity of many managed care regulations. A psychiatrist's office, for instance, telephoned an insurance company regarding coverage for a girl who had been sexually abused. The office was told, "Sexual abuse is worth 15 sessions—but if it's incest, she gets 20." Is it any wonder that doctors feel inclined to game this system? Reimbursement rules that do not cover the actual needs of patients make gaming the system tempting for the physician who wishes to act in the patient's best interest. Gaming the system is also tempting for the physician wishing to line his or her pockets by performing unnecessary and profitable procedures.

The trouble is, gaming the system is also fraud. However well-intentioned it may be, it can easily slide into even worse fraud, where physicians and other providers manipulate reimbursement rules for their own gain. In one recent and well-reported example, cardiologists at Redding Medical Center in northern California were charged with performing unnecessary heart procedures on Medicare patients, and their employer wound up settling the case for $54 million (Associated Press 2004). Medical fraud is estimated to cost

Americans tens of billions, if not hundreds of billions, of dollars. Some part of that total includes physicians who lie and cheat to get what their patients need, as well as those who lie and cheat to line their own pockets.

Fraud is only one example of the fact that doctors are human beings with all of a human being's frailties. Some physicians have drug or alcohol problems. Some have difficult personalities: they yell at their associates, they are brusque or abrupt with their patients, they bridle at rules and regulations designed to protect patients. Some engage in sexual harassment. A small minority of doctors are simply inept or incompetent; about 5 percent of physicians are responsible for more than 50 percent of malpractice awards, and the average award is about $4 million (Mello and Hemenway 2004). Like fraud, all these behaviors contribute to an erosion of trust, particularly because doctors are unwilling to blow the whistle on their colleagues.

So while the public generally holds physicians in high esteem, not all of people's attitudes toward doctors are positive. About half of the public agrees with the statement, "Doctors are not as thorough as they should be." About half—no more—agree that "Doctors always treat patients with respect." And 41 percent believe that "Doctors cause people to worry a lot because they don't explain medical problems to patients" (National Opinion Research Center 1998).

MEDICAL RESEARCH

A third issue that threatens the public's trust in individual providers—a major trustbuster—is the conduct of scientific research in medicine and, in particular, human subjects research.

Medical advice is always imperfect. When doctors tell their patients what to take, what to eat, and how to take care of themselves, they are necessarily relying on accumulated scientific information produced by research. Inevitably, some of this research is proven wrong by subsequent research. For example, physicians for years advised menopausal women to pursue a regimen of hormone replacement therapy, and some 20 million women in the United States followed their advice. Since July 2002, however, many of these women have discontinued the therapy; new research shows that it involves more long-term risks than benefits (Rossouw et al. 2002). When medical advice changes, people react in a variety of ways, often self-defeating. Many lose trust in their physicians. Many others decide that healthcare professionals in general do not know what they are talking about, so you might as well do anything you want.

Behind the apparent flip-flops is another trust-related issue: how the research that produces advances in scientific knowledge is conducted. Human subjects research involves large-scale experiments, typically following a standard "double blind" protocol. A group of patients with a given condition is identified. Half of the patients are given an experimental new medicine, the other half a placebo. Neither the patients nor their physicians know who has received which. Trust is obviously an essential element of this procedure, as physicians and healthcare leaders well understand. Former Secretary of Health and Human Services Donna Shalala (2000) wrote, "...if we are to keep testing new medicines and new approaches to curing disease, we cannot compromise the trust and willingness of patients to participate in clinical trials." An article in the journal *Archives of Internal Medicine* put the matter even more bluntly (Kahn and Mastroianni 2001):

> The success of clinical research lies in the element of trust—trust in researchers, trust in hospitals, and trust in the research process itself.... Without trust at all these levels, research could not be carried out. Potential subjects would be unwilling to put themselves in harm's way if they perceived that they would be used by researchers, institutions, or those who fund research, and society at large would be unwilling to have its dollars spent on an enterprise that neither enjoyed nor deserved its trust.

The trouble is, the research process has *not* earned the public's trust and is therefore in jeopardy. Consider two of the key issues—informed consent and financial incentives—discussed below.

Informed Consent

No one is allowed to participate in a clinical trial without signing a piece of paper saying that they understand and agree to the terms of the experiment—that is, they give their informed consent. The process of gaining consent, however, differs from study to study; investigators are given wide latitude in enrolling research subjects. There is also a scarcity of documentation concerning what people actually understand when they agree to be subjects of new drug or vaccine trials. What little research there is indicates that people sometimes fail to grasp that they are in an experiment; that the drug they (may) receive is not proven to help, and may in fact worsen their health; and that they may not receive the drug at all, but rather a placebo. This lack of understanding undermines the whole notion of informed consent.

Financial Incentives

Physicians who enroll their patients in clinical trials are compensated by the drug company or agency that is conducting the research. The amount of the funds involved can be significant, and patients may be unaware of the fact that their doctor is receiving money for participating in the research. At times, physicians may even have a financial interest in the pharmaceutical company that manufactures the experimental drug. This raises all the issues inherent in the principal-agent relationship discussed earlier. Patients assume that the physician is their agent, but physicians are often acting on behalf of researchers and in their own interests.

In the past, patients went along with all kinds of research, some of it wholly unethical, just because their doctors suggested it. The committee investigating the human radiation experiments conducted by the federal government between 1944 and 1974, for instance, heard responses such as these (Advisory Committee on Human Radiation Experiments 1995):

> They know what they're doing. They wouldn't have you do this if they didn't know what they were doing.
>
> He asked me if I wanted to go on it, and I said, "If it's what you think I should do, yes, because you know more about it than I do..."
>
> To me, they are the doctors, and once I had gotten those doctors and I trusted them...it was pretty much up to them.

Today, however, the tide of trust is turning. Asked to rate their confidence in various aspects of medical research, poll respondents expressed significant doubts about researchers' trustworthiness. Only about one-quarter were "very confident" that new treatments were tested on humans only after there was valid scientific evidence that the treatments are likely to be safe and effective. About the same number were very confident that patients are told "honestly and clearly" about the risks involved—and that patients "are treated as patients, not as guinea pigs." Only 20 percent were very confident that money was *not* the driving factor in recruiting patients, and only 13 percent were very confident that patients would not suffer more pain or side-effects than they would from standard treatment (Harris Interactive 2002).

Distrust of healthcare providers in general may also make some people less likely to trust the results of clinical trials.

MORE THAN HALF EMPTY

A few years ago, a group of researchers asked focus groups composed of African-American patients what came to mind when they heard the term "medical research." Many of the responses were harsh. In the "trust" category, for instance, respondents came up with phrases such as "being lied to," "corruption," "deception," and "negligence." The term "guinea pig" occurred repeatedly: one participant in the study said, "They always use our race as a guinea pig"; another said,

"They treat us like guinea pigs. They are trying stuff out on us—stuff they learned in school" (Corbie-Smith et al. 1999).

A more recent study compared responses from African-Americans and whites to several questions relating to human subjects research. By large margins, African-American respondents were less likely to trust that their physicians would fully explain research participation to them, were more likely to believe that their physicians might expose them to unnecessary risks, and were more likely to believe that their physicians had *already* given them treatment as part of an experiment without their permission. On a seven-item index of distrust compiled by the researchers, African Americans scored significantly higher than whites (3.1 to 1.8). Race remained a highly significant variable even when the researchers controlled for other social and demographic variables specifically correlated with high distrust (Corbie-Smith, Thomas, and St. George 2002).[2]

In this case, distrust of medical research is but the tip of a large iceberg, namely, a lack of trust in healthcare in general among many members of low-income and minority populations. (As noted in Chapter 2, the *erosion* of trust has affected all groups of Americans more or less equally, but the *level* of trust—the starting point—varies from group to group.) The lack of trust is seen most clearly, and is best documented, among people of color, but it is by no means limited to these populations.

- Fifteen percent of African Americans, 13 percent of Hispanics, and 11 percent of Asian Americans believe that they would receive better healthcare if they were of different race or ethnicity, compared to only 1 percent of whites (Collins et al. 2002).[3]
- Among insured Americans, only 66.8 percent of African Americans and 70.8 percent of Hispanics have a regular healthcare provider, compared with 78.1 percent of whites; among the uninsured, the corresponding figures are 18.4 percent for African Americans, 20.3 percent for Hispanics, and 51.4 percent for whites (Hargraves 2002). We know that trust is a strong predictor of patient loyalty to a physician; data such

as these would seem to indicate a lack of trust (National Research Corporation 2002).

- Racial and ethnic minorities are almost twice as concerned as the general population about errors when they receive healthcare (Kaiser Family Foundation/Agency for Healthcare Research and Quality 2000).
- Recent immigrants may experience trust-related issues of their own. An immigrant from Russia may expect to bribe a doctor to get the medicine he needs. A pregnant woman from Korea may want a little seaweed soup to get over an ailment. Many Asian immigrants may be put off by direct eye contact and a firm handshake from the doctor. Failure to understand such cultural differences may undermine trust in even a well-meaning clinician.

Trust in individual providers is threatened not only by systemwide phenomena but also by disparities in the treatment people receive from healthcare professionals—and by their perception that they are being given short shrift.

NOTES

1. A total of 23 professions were ranked. The historical average of medical doctors who rated high or very high in esteem between 1976 and 2003 is 56 percent.
2. The seven-item index consists of the following questions:
   —If your physician wanted you to participate in research, do you trust that he or she would fully explain it to you? (disagree or do not know)
   —Do you believe that you can freely ask your physicians any questions you want? (no or do not know)
   —Your physician would not ask you to participate in medical research if he or she thought it would harm you. (disagree or do not know)

—In deciding what treatments you will get, do you feel that your physicians always try to protect you from unnecessary risk, or do you feel that they sometimes expose you to unnecessary risk? (expose to unnecessary risk or do not know)
—How likely is it that you, or people like you, might be used as guinea pigs without your consent? (very likely, somewhat likely, or do not know)
—How often, if ever, do you think physicians prescribe medication as a way of experimenting on people without their knowledge or consent? (very often, fairly often, or do not know)
—Do you believe that physicians have ever given you treatment as part of an experiment without your permission? (yes or do not know)

3. Sample included 3,488 whites, 1,152 Hispanics, 1,037 African Americans, and 669 Asian Americans.

REFERENCES

Advisory Committee on Human Radiation Experiments. 1995. *Final Report of the Advisory Committee on Human Radiation Experiments*. Subject No. 332324-2 (3/24/95 lines 309–11); Subject No. 552264-4 (3/14/95 lines 194–98); Subject No. 114250-4 (3/10/95 lines 274–83). Washington, DC: U.S. Government Printing Office.

Associated Press. 2004. "Tenet Healthcare in Talks to Settle Probes." *Boston Globe* June 13, E3.

Break the Chain. http://www.breakthechain.org/exclusives/drguns.html.

Brennan, T. A., L. L. Leape, N. M. Laird, L. Herbert, A. R. Localio, A. G. Lawthers, J. P. Newhouse, et al. 1991. "Incidence of Adverse Events and Negligence in Hospitalized Patients: Results of the Harvard Medical Practice Study I." *New England Journal of Medicine* 324: 370–76.

Collins, K. S., D. L. Hughes, M. M. Doty, B. L. Ives, J. N. Edwards, and K. Tenney. 2002. *Diverse Communities, Common Concerns: Assessing Health Care Quality for Minority Americans: Findings from the Commonwealth Fund 2001 Health Care Quality Survey*, 30, 33. [Online report; retrieved 11/17/04.] http://www.cmwf.org /usr_doc/collins_diversecommun_523.pdf.

Corbie-Smith, G., S. B. Thomas, and D. M. St. George. 2002. "Distrust, Race and Research." *Archives of Internal Medicine* 162 (21): 2458–63.

Corbie-Smith, G., S. B. Thomas, M. V. Williams, and S. Moody-Ayers. 1999. "Attitudes and Beliefs of African-Americans Toward Participation in Medical Research." *Journal of General Internal Medicine* 14 (9): 540.

Crawshaw, R., D. E. Rogers, E. D. Pellegrino, R. J. Bulger, G. D. Lundberg, L. R. Bristow, C. K. Cassel, and J. A. Barondess. 1995. "Patient-Physician Covenant." *Journal of the American Medical Association* 273 (19): 1553.

Elliott, V. S. 2002. "Drug Diluting in Kansas City: A Pharmacist's Crime Shakes a Community." *Amamednews.com*. http://www.ama-assn.org/amednews/2002/05/20/hll10520.htm.

Gallup News Service. 2003. "Public Rates Nursing as Most Honest and Ethical Profession." Dec. 1. [Online information; retrieved 11/17/04.] http://www.gallup.com/content/default.aspx?ci=9823&pg=1.

Hargraves, J. L. 2002. "The Insurance Gap and Minority Health Care, 1997–2001." [Online information; retrieved 11/17/04.] http://www.hschange.org/CONTENT/443/.

Harris Interactive. 2002. "There Are Many Reasons Why People Are Reluctant to Participate in Clinical Trials." *Health Care News* 2 (7): 2–3.

Kahn, J. P., and A. C. Mastroianni. 2001. "Moving from Compliance to Conscience: Why We Can and Should Improve on the Ethics of Clinical Research." *Archives of Internal Medicine* 161 (7): 925–28.

Kaiser Family Foundation/Agency for Healthcare Research and Quality. 2000. *National Survey on Americans as Healthcare Consumers: An Update on the Role of Quality Information*. Menlo Park, CA: Kaiser Family Foundation and the Agency for Healthcare Research and Quality.

Kocieniewski, D. 2004. "Ex-Nurse Pleads Guilty to Killing Patients." *New York Times* April 30, B1.

Kohn, L. T., J. M. Corrigan, and M. Donaldson. 2000. *To Err Is Human: Building a Safer Health System*. Institute of Medicine. Washington, DC: National Academies Press.

Mello, M. M., and D. Hemenway. 2004. "Medical Malpractice as an Epidemiological Problem." *Social Science & Medicine* 59 (1): 39–46.

National Opinion Research Center. 1998. *U.S. General Social Survey*. Chicago: University of Chicago.

National Research Corporation. 2002."What Determines Patient Loyalty: The Top Factors." In *National Research Corporation Performance Tool Kit,* vol. 2, p. 1.

[Online information; retrieved 11/17/04.] http://www.nationalresearch.com /toolkit/Feb2002Toolkit.pdf.

Rossouw, J. E., et al. 2002. "Risks and Benefits of Estrogen Plus Progestin in Healthly Postmenopausal Women: Principal Results for the Women's Health Initiative Randomized Controlled Trial." *Journal of the American Medical Association* 288 (3): 321–33.

Shalala, D. 2000. "Protecting Research Subjects—What Must Be Done." *New England Journal of Medicine* 343 (11): 809.

Starfield, B. 2000. "Is U.S. Health Really the Best in the World?" *Journal of the American Medical Association* 284 (4): 483–85.

Steinhauer, J., and E. Wong. 2000. "How Doctor Got Work After Carving Into Patient." *New York Times* Jan. 27, 81.

Wynia, M. K., D. S. Cummings, J. B. VanGeest, and I. B. Wilson. 2000. "Physician Manipulation of Reimbursement Rules for Patients Between a Rock and a Hard Place." *Journal of the American Medical Association* 283 (14): 1861.

CHAPTER FOUR

Healthcare Hype and Other Influences

No man is an island, entire of itself...

—John Donne

JUST AS NO man or woman is an island, neither is any healthcare provider. Doctors and nurses, hospitals and managed care organizations, pharmaceutical companies and nursing homes all operate in a kind of societywide fishbowl. Virtually everything they do is subject to scrutiny and a potential topic for criticism or approbation. Everyone has opinions about medical care, so it seems, and few are hesitant to express them. Healthcare is an unusual industry in many ways; one difference between healthcare and everything else is that it is uniquely public.

This fact has dramatic ramifications for the subject of trust. While the last two chapters have focused on what happens inside healthcare—on the trust issues that healthcare organizations and providers confront directly in their work—we turn now to what happens outside healthcare, in the larger society. This chapter and the next offer brief surveys of how other institutions and constituencies—the media, governments, consumers themselves—have contributed to the erosion of trust in healthcare. As we will see in Part II of the book, understanding this public aspect of the trust crisis is critically important to understanding the trust prescription. It is not enough simply to build trust; providers and organizations must come to be *known* for trust. They must establish not just a trust capacity but also a public reputation based on trust. If they can do so, they can begin to reverse the spiral of distrust described in these chapters.

BAD NEWS FROM THE MEDIA

The headlines about healthcare that greet newspaper readers and television viewers these days are often raucous and frightening. Consider the following:

- "Betrayal of Trust: The Collapse of Global Public Health"
- "Patients Trust Doctors but Suspicious of Healthcare System"
- "A Hospital's Conflict of Interest: Patients Weren't Told of Stake in Cancer Drug"
- "Building Trust Before It's Too Late"

Given such headlines, it would be easy to blame the entire trust crisis in healthcare on fear-mongering by the media. But to attribute the crisis to the media alone would be to blame the messenger for their own failings. That said, the media exacerbate the crisis in a variety of ways. It is worth going beyond the scary headlines to see exactly what newspapers, television, and other media do and why they do it. As we will see, their role is both complex and influential.

The most visible impact of the media lies in the stories that announce an error, a foul-up, a financial crisis, or some other disaster. Healthcare organizations naturally dread such pieces, and most devote considerable attention to keeping whatever bad news they may generate out of the paper (or at least portrayed in the most favorable light possible). The "perfect storm" for this kind of situation probably occurred a few years ago, when *Boston Globe* health reporter Betsy Lehman died from a medication error administered at Dana Farber Cancer Center (Allen 1995). Such mistakes, as we have seen, happen with distressing frequency in American hospitals. When they happen to a staff member of the city's most prominent newspaper—and a healthcare reporter to boot—the institution can assume that the story will be pursued relentlessly and given wide play. That, of course, is precisely what happened.

The hard-news departments of major newspapers and television stations *always* trade on, and look for, bad news of this sort. The fact that most of a hospital's patients are treated successfully and go home happy or that a managed care organization pays nearly all its bills and keeps nearly all of its members and providers happy is not worth their attention. The stories that hit the morning's headlines or the nightly news will necessarily be negative: the medication errors in hospitals, the unnecessary deaths in nursing homes, the patients left unattended in the emergency room, the family denied coverage by its insurance company. When the Boston-area surgeon left a patient in the operating room to attend to some business at his bank, the event was as rare as it was outrageous. Never mind; that particular story instantly went out over a thousand wires and airwaves. It is just such pieces, media experts tell us, that their readers and viewers want to see.

The cumulative effect of these bad-news articles creates a kind of illusion in the mind of the news consumer. The illusion is that such events are happening all the time. Just as crime stories engender the feeling that the streets are more and more dangerous—even when crime rates are dropping—"medical disaster" stories lead people to think that you can never be too careful in the healthcare system. They encourage people to believe that you cannot trust anybody.

FLIP-FLOPS

Another sort of story that invariably makes news is the reversal of some sort of health-related or conventional medical advice. I mentioned the apparent flip-flop relating to hormone replacement therapy in the previous chapter—just one among many reversals of medical advice traceable to new knowledge. The area that often hits closest to home for ordinary consumers is public health, and recommendations about diet in particular. Should you eat butter or margarine? Are eggs really bad for you? Should you eat more carbohydrates or fewer? The conflicting advice to be found in the media on such matters would fill volumes, not to mention the vast amount of additional material supporting each side that can be turned up on the Internet. Who can be trusted? Here, too, according to the reports in the media, a reasonable conclusion would be, "no one."

Even the government is not immune from contradiction. For years, the U.S. Department of Agriculture food pyramid has served as the official summary of the government's advice about how many daily servings of various foods should be included in a healthy diet. The pyramid has appeared on the back of cereal boxes and milk cartons. It is taught in the schools. It was considered to be the gold standard of dietary advice, backed with the imprimatur of the U.S. government. Yet my colleague Walter Willett (2005) and his associates have concluded, based on a series of studies, that the advice contained in the pyramid could be considered misleading and perhaps even wrong. It makes no distinction between different types of carbohydrates, for example, even though whole grains such as whole wheat and brown rice are far more healthful than refined or "white" products. It makes no distinction between different types of fats and oils, even though research shows that some kinds of fats are far more healthful than others.

HEALTHCARE HYPE

There is, of course, another kind of story entirely that regularly appears in the media: the "soft news" health-related feature. Typically, these stories highlight a new drug, a new test, or a new procedure. They usually tell the heartwarming story of a patient who had given up hope but was helped by the new development. People in the media call these "feel good" stories, because the aim is not to expose but to comfort. The hidden message is, "There may be help for you, too."

But as award-winning health journalist Trudy Lieberman of Consumers Union has pointed out, these articles often suffer from two kinds of problems. One is a certain breathless quality: the new test or treatment is suddenly the answer to everybody's problems. There is little consideration of when the new test or treatment might be appropriate and when it might not be. When ThinPrep was introduced, for instance—ThinPrep is a new way of testing for cervical cancer through Pap smears—reporters rarely asked the critically important question of how many false positives the new technique generated. Without that information it was difficult for consumers to judge the pros and cons of using it.

A second problem is that of potential conflicts of interest. Media companies may be owned by larger corporate entities with a business interest in healthcare, and a possible influence on news stories.

While readers and viewers may enjoy seeing such stories, they may learn in time that many of the articles are not to be wholly trusted. In this way, too, the media help to undermine trust in the healthcare system.

THE POWER OF TELEVISION...

When researchers study the effect of the media on a field such as healthcare, they typically focus (as I have just done) on news articles. But fictional dramas created for prime-time television represent at least as much influence. If news is the text of our culture, then these are the subtext. And what a change we have witnessed in this arena. If you are old enough, you will remember the kindly, trustworthy Marcus Welby, M.D., or perhaps the bold and handsome Dr. Kildare. Back then, TV physicians were made out to be heroes.

Today, some physicians are still portrayed as heroes, such as (most of) the doctors on the popular show *ER*. But the picture of healthcare as a whole on today's television dramas is both more complex and considerably less positive. According to a study conducted for the Kaiser Family Foundation, for instance, TV medical dramas featured an average of one scene per episode that discussed a public policy healthcare issue (Turow and Gans 2002). Examples include the following:

- An episode of a popular Lifetime show, *Strong Medicine*, in which a critically ill low-income patient does not have access to the prescription drugs she needs because her inner-city neighborhood is not adequately served by the major pharmacies (Thus do issues such as disparities of care, mentioned in the previous chapter, make their way into the public consciousness.)
- A story on the (now-canceled) ABC drama *Gideon's Crossing* about a woman whose leukemia was misdiagnosed by her overworked and possibly careless HMO doctor
- An *ER* episode in which an HMO will not allow a woman with terminal breast cancer to be admitted to a hospital for pain management

The Kaiser study concluded that the shows did not tilt either for or against the status quo of healthcare in their depictions of these health issues. But they did frequently reference many of the leading institutional players in health policy debates, including hospital administrators, lawyers, government agencies, insurance companies, and HMOs. Of these, insurance companies, lawyers, and HMOs were portrayed more negatively than positively. (Indeed, every single reference to HMOs during the 2000–2001 television season was negative. While the study found that the depiction of healthcare was balanced overall, the six situations depicting HMOs were all portrayed negatively. [Turow and Gans 2002].)

Any given news story is likely to be read or viewed by fewer than a million people. Prime-time television, by contrast, is typically watched by tens of millions. Moreover, the dramas are likely to be more powerfully presented than the news shows. "Instead of bill numbers and budget figures," says Vicky Rideout, vice president of the Kaiser Family Foundation, "health policy issues are portrayed through the lives of characters the viewer cares about, often in life or death situations" (Kaiser Family Foundation 2002a). The dramas conjure up a visceral reaction in the viewer that reinforces whatever cognitive mistrust has been generated by news stories.

...AND THE BIG SCREEN

An even more powerful medium than television, of course, is the Hollywood feature film, and where healthcare is concerned, no film may be more powerful than *John Q*, released in 2002 by New Line Cinema. The movie's protagonist is John Q. Archibald, played by Denzel Washington. Archibald's son, Michael, needs a heart transplant, and Archibald is shocked and horrified to learn that his insurance company does not cover the procedure. Meanwhile, the hospital that will perform the transplant is demanding $75,000 in advance, which Archibald does not have. The story is about the desperate measures he takes to try to get the medical care his son needs to survive.

This movie is based on a true story—a real-life David versus Goliath saga—and Archibald is one of the more sympathetic characters to grace the big screen in recent memory. The story begins, moreover, with a flagrant contradiction that nearly every moviegoer can relate to. Archibald *has* health insurance. His son *needs* an expensive procedure. Why would anyone have insurance *except* to cover situations like this? Why would any insurance policy *not* cover a lifesaving procedure? What is going on here, anyway? The movie is an extraordinary indictment of the U.S. healthcare system, and it is told, like the television dramas, at a deeply emotional level. It also hit a raw nerve. Between 12 million and 15 million people saw *John Q* in theaters, and millions more have seen it on videotape and DVD. Among those who had heard of the movie, more than seven in ten said they believe insurers refused to pay for treatments like those portrayed; 42 percent believe this happens "a lot," while 30 percent believe it happens "sometimes" (Kaiser Family Foundation 2002b). In response to the film, the American Association of Health Plans (AAHP) announced in summer 2002 that it had retained Hollywood's leading talent agency, William Morris, in an attempt to "build bridges between health plans and the entertainment community." In other words, the AAHP would like Hollywood to portray HMOs and insurance companies more favorably. But the prognosis was not good. Just about the time that the AAHP was making its overtures, the Showtime network offered a movie called *Damaged Care,* a fictionalized account of a real-life managed care executive who went on to become an outspoken critic of the industry. ABC announced a new medical drama that would feature two renegade doctors trying to take on (what else?) HMOs.

PERCEPTION VERSUS REALITY

In some fields, people's attitudes are independent of what actually happens. Devout sports fans may wish, hope, and pray for their team's victory, but the team will either win or lose depending on how well it plays relative to the other team. Trust in healthcare is different. To be sure, people's first-hand experiences with the healthcare system affect trust levels. But so, too, do a host of other factors, including anecdotes from friends and relatives, news stories, and dramatic accounts of healthcare crises. Where trust is concerned, perception is not only affected by reality, it *is* reality.

This fact intensifies the trust crisis in healthcare for two reasons. First, not everything that affects trust is under the control of healthcare professionals. Hospitals, physicians, HMOs, and nursing homes might all simultaneously improve their performance on the many different scales that affect trust. But another movie as popular and as powerful as *John Q*—or a report on *60 Minutes*, say, about a serious but isolated problem in one facet of the healthcare system—could undermine all that effort in a heartbeat. Ultimately, changes in reality do affect what people read in the media and how they react to those stories. But where a sports fan's attitude may change quickly, depending only on a stretch of victories or defeats, a healthcare consumer's attitudes will change only slowly.

Second, there is a phenomenon in measurement known as *response shift* that powerfully affects trust levels. Response shifts occur over time as expectations change based on new information and experiences. For instance, if we expect a 30-minute wait in the doctor's office and we experience wait times of only 15 minutes for several appointments, not only may we be pleasantly surprised but our expectation is also likely to shift: we expect that the wait time in the future will only be 15 minutes. If, after that shift takes place, the doctor takes 30 minutes to see us, we will be disappointed and angry. So it is with healthcare in general. Our levels of trust depend greatly on our expectations. We respond to reports and stories in the media based on our expectations as well. As expectations change, we may continue to feel mistrustful over events that once might have seemed acceptable. After all, before heart transplants became as common as they are, John Q. Archibald's outrage would have seemed quixotic. Today, we have come to believe that Archibald's son—or anybody else with health insurance, maybe anybody else at all—is entitled to a heart transplant. If the transplant is not forthcoming, we lose trust in the healthcare system.

So the dimensions of the trust crisis are widened and hardened by the media. By shaping perceptions, they deepen consumers' mistrust. Not surprisingly, consumers have reacted. They feel vulnerable, and they have begun to take matters into their own hands.

REFERENCES

Allen, S. 1995. "Elite Cancer Center Gave Journalist Fatal Drug Dose." *Modern Healthcare* March 27, 9.

Kaiser Family Foundation. 2002a. "Television Hospital Dramas Often Draw on Public Policy Debated for Story Lines, Study Says." Daily Health Policy Report: Media and Society. July 17. [Online information; retrieved] http://www.kaisernet-work.org/daily_reports /rep_index.cfm?hint=38dr_id=12370.

Kaiser Family Foundation. 2002b. "Response to the Movie John Q." Survey conducted as part of the Health News Interest Index series, released at the forum *John Q Goes to Washington: Health Policy Issues in Popular Culture,* Washington, DC, July 16.

Lieberman, T. 2005. "Trustworthy Information: The Role of the Media." In *The Trust Crisis in Healthcare: Causes, Consequences and Cures*, edited by D. A. Shore. New York: Oxford University Press.

Turow, J., and R. Gans 2002. *As Seen on TV: Health Policy Issues in TV's Medical Dramas.* Report to the Kaiser Family Foundation. [Online report; retrieved 11/17/04.] http://www.kff.org/entmedia/John_Q_Report.pdf.

Willett, W. C. 2005. "Confusion at the Table: Can We Trust that Our Food Is Healthy?" In *The Trust Crisis in Healthcare: Causes, Consequences and Cures,* edited by D. A. Shore. New York: Oxford University Press.

CHAPTER FIVE

What Happens When Trust Erodes?

Skepticism is slow suicide.

—*Ralph Waldo Emerson*

TRUST AND VULNERABILITY go hand in hand: when people feel vulnerable, they experience a greater need for trust. That is why trust in the federal government leaped right after the attack on Pearl Harbor in 1941 and again after September 11, 2001. But there is a self-reinforcing loop in this equation. A *lack* of trust increases feelings of vulnerability, which creates a greater need for trust, and so on. The upshot of this negative spiral is that the trust crisis in healthcare cannot simply be ignored. If healthcare organizations and professionals do not take it on, consumers themselves will do so. Nobody wants to feel vulnerable in the face of illness or injury, and if people sense that they cannot trust the healthcare system, they will try to change things so that they can. To protect themselves, they will seek out or create trust *surrogates*. The two most common of these are government regulation and consumer activism.

This phenomenon can be seen clearly in the 1970s, when the last trust famine occurred (see box). For a variety of reasons, trust in government, business, and a number of other institutions plummeted during that decade. It was also the decade of the first great round of consumer activism and government regulation in the modern era. Ralph Nader and his supporters gained prominence. The environmental movement grew to be influential nationwide. Federal agencies such as the Occupational Safety and Health Administration were born. Such waves of regulation reflect the paradox: we need to trust because we feel vulnerable, but we do not trust, so we feel still more vulnerable. To make the system more trustworthy, we impose requirements to encourage or force better behavior. But whether this actually builds trust or undermines it is far from clear.

THE NEW WAVE OF REGULATION

It is exactly this paradox that can be seen today in the plethora of legislative proposals and efforts toward self-regulation in the healthcare industry. Among them are report cards, the Health Insurance Portability and Accountability Act (HIPAA), and a number of operational regulations, as discussed in the following sections.

Institutional and Individual Report Cards

How does hospital A stack up against hospitals B, C, D, and E? How do the managed care plans available in California or Connecticut compare with their competitors? How do Chicago-area nursing homes compare with one another on a series of measures? If reliable information on such matters were available, the rationale behind report cards goes, we would know which institutions we could trust, and we would encourage organizations to build up their trust capacity. Much the same thinking applies to individual providers. How many kidney transplant operations has a particular surgeon done? What is his or her success rate? What are the disciplinary records of every doctor on my health plan? Which physicians are rated highest by their patients, and which are rated lowest?

The Last Trust Famine

The first great wave of regulation and consumerism to hit healthcare occurred in the 1970s. At that time, the federal government first began requiring large employers to offer their employees a managed care alternative to traditional insurance plans. And what lay behind the wave? A sharp decline in public trust—in all areas.

The numbers tell the story. Trust in the federal government plummeted from 76 percent in 1964 to 36 percent in 1974 and to 25 percent by 1980 (National Election Studies 1995–2000). Trust in major companies fell from 55 percent in 1966 to 16 percent in 1980 (Taylor 2003). Confidence in the leaders of medicine fell from 73 percent in 1966 to 34 percent in 1980 (Harris Poll). Even interpersonal trust fell sharply. The number of people agreeing with the statement, "Most other people can be trusted" stood at 46 percent in 1972; by 1980 it was down to 37 percent (Davis 1972–1994).

Sources: Gallup Poll; Yankelovich Surveys and Gallup Poll; Harris Poll; Washington Post, Kaiser, and Harvard University Poll.

Davis, J. A. 1972–1994. *General Social Survey Cumulative File*. Chicago: National Opinion Research Center.

National Election Studies. 1995–2000.

Taylor, H. 2003. "While Confidence in Leaders and Institutions Has Dropped from the Extraordinary Post-9/11 High, it Is Still Higher than it Was for Most of the Late 70s, 80s, and 90s." *The Harris Poll* #4. [Online article; retrieved 1/22/03.] http://www.harrisinteractive.com/harris_poll/index.asp?PID=351.

One such report card is the state of California's assessment of HMOs. California rates health plans using the well-known Health Plan Employer Data and Information Set (HEDIS) and Consumer Assessment of Health Plans Survey (CAHPS) performance ratings. Both ratings systems survey randomly selected samples of plan members to assess whether they received particular services indicated by their medical conditions (HEDIS) and how they rated their overall experiences with the plans (CAHPS). Summary quality scores run from "excellent" to "poor" and assess plan performance in categories such as "care for staying healthy," "care for getting better," and "doctor communication and services."

Outside of California, however, not many such report cards have been issued, and the few that do exist have provoked enormous controversy. Some of the controversy reflects real difficulties in measuring quality. For example, hospitals that routinely treat older or sicker patients may report above-average death rates, but no one wants to penalize them for treating these patients. Some of the controversy also reflects organizational and individual self-interest. Few providers or provider organizations enjoy having their records on display for public scrutiny. So the political objections to any kind of comprehensive public reporting system are formidable.

HIPAA

The Health Insurance Portability and Accountability Act, passed in 1996, enacted a number of reforms, such as ensuring that workers moving from one employer to another can enjoy uninterrupted health insurance coverage. It also included a number of provisions relating to the privacy and confidentiality of patients' medical records.

HIPAA reflected some very real concerns about the information these records contain. What exactly is in them? Before HIPAA, patients in 16 states did not even have the right to see their medical records. Will the records be kept confidential? Will the information they contain somehow be used against me, for example, by my employer? Patients are particularly skittish about the privacy of mental health records. HIPAA includes a "notice" section requiring that patients must now be informed about what is happening to their data and that they have access to their records. They have the right to request amendments to their records and the right to request restrictions on disclosure of the information. Healthcare organizations are liable for substantial penalties if they violate HIPAA standards. In preparation for the law's effective date—April 14, 2003—healthcare organizations found that they had to devote considerable resources to ensuring compliance with HIPAA's provisions.

Operational Regulations

A bellwether law in California, passed in 1999 and scheduled to be implemented over a period of years, mandates nurse-to-patient ratios in hospitals for the stated purpose of reducing errors in care and burnout among nurses. Before the law was passed, minimum nurse ratios were already in place in respiratory care, coronary care, and well-baby units, as well as in operating rooms; the law extended the requirement to all other parts of the hospital, including medical/surgical wards. California mandated that hospitals must have at least one nurse for every six medical or surgical patients by January 2004 and one for every five by 2005. When the law is fully implemented, no unit will have fewer than one nurse for every eight patients. Current staffing recommendations vary from three to ten patients per nurse.

This law reflects the acute anxiety—and loss of trust—that consumers feel when they read headlines such as "Nursing Shortage Can Have Deadly Consequences," or statistics such as those (mentioned earlier) that appeared in 2002 in the *Journal of the American Medical Association (JAMA)*. According to the *JAMA* article, the risk of dying after surgery jumps 14 percent when a patient's nurse has six beds to cover rather than four and soars by more than 30 percent if the nurse is responsible for eight beds. Put another way, a hospital with six patients per nurse rather than four could expect 2.3 additional deaths and nearly 9 additional complications per 1,000 patients. With a ratio of eight to one, there would be 2.6 more deaths and almost 10 more complications for every thousand (Aiken et al. 2002). Of course, the California law is hugely controversial. Nurses' organizations and public-employee unions support it, whereas hospitals fiercely oppose it. Given the nationwide nursing shortage, moreover—a shortage that is particularly acute in California—it is not clear where healthcare providers will find the additional nurses they will need to comply with the law. Nor is it clear how effectively the state will enforce the new regulations. "In the 27 years since California first instituted staffing ratios for a select set of intensive care units," reports the *Sacramento Bee* (2003), "state officials have not issued a single fine for violations."

Assessment and regulation, actual and proposed, hardly stop with these examples. The Leapfrog Group, a coalition of employers founded by the Business Roundtable, provides information about hospital performance in an attempt to improve quality and reduce medical errors. The Joint Commission on Accreditation of Healthcare Organizations has proposed voluntary guidelines for disclosure of errors. The National Committee for Quality Assurance accredits managed care plans based on the plans' HEDIS scores. Meanwhile, interest in a national patients' bill of rights seems to ebb and flow. In 2001, thanks to a "surprise deal" between the Bush administration and Rep. Charles Whitlow Norwood (R-Ga), the leading congressional proponent of patients' rights, it seemed likely that Congress would pass legislation. As of June 22, 2004, ten states have passed patients' bills of rights, but as this book goes to press, the issue has more or less faded away in Washington, in part because state legislators, courts, and the managed care industry have themselves taken measures to protect patients' rights (Goldstein 2003).

All of this reflects a decline of trust, yet all of it may ultimately help to build trust. The old Turkish proverb, "Trust in Allah, but tie up your camel"—adapted by Ronald Reagan as "Trust, but verify"—is applicable in healthcare. Even the most skeptical of patients may feel reassured when more information is available and when government agencies or industry organizations are helping to enforce standards.

THE NEW CONSUMERISM

Consumerism usually refers to advocacy by organized groups working on behalf of consumers' interests. There is some of that in healthcare, but the consumerist attitude today usually takes other forms. Chief among these is the belief on the part of consumers that they must manage their own healthcare. In the past, patients typically showed up at a doctor's office, described a complaint or two, and took whatever prescriptions or treatments the doctor suggested. In the past, too, they showed up at hospitals whenever their doctor recommended a hospital-based procedure, and they did whatever the hospital staff instructed them to do, without question. Today, as every healthcare provider knows, many patients take a wholly different approach. They express opinions about the nature of their complaints and about what an appropriate treatment might be. They ask questions that they never would have asked in the past. They challenge the advice and orders of medical professionals: Why is this necessary? Why are you suggesting that? What are the alternatives?

The healthcare model has been altered dramatically. It used to be based on *compliance*; the physician was in charge, and the patient was expected to comply. Over time it moved closer to *adherence*; the physician was still in charge, but the patient voluntarily adhered closely to the doctor's recommendations. Today, for many patients, it might best be described as *concordance*. Neither party dominates the relationship. The patient is no longer passive; he or she seeks to be an active partner. This is particularly true in the case of chronic diseases, where patients have time to educate themselves and a substantial interest in doing so. In some instances, physicians have told me, their relationship with chronic patients is very much like a relationship between two professionals, with each party having more or less equal knowledge of the alternatives.

Why has the relationship changed so dramatically? The list of causal factors is long, but at a minimum it includes those discussed in the following paragraphs.

Patients are more educated and less intimidated. Education levels have been rising throughout the United States. As they do, the proportion of people who feel intimidated by medical authority or medical language diminishes. Most college graduates believe they know enough to understand the basics of what a physician tells them. They ask for explanations, whereas their less-educated counterparts in the past would simply have taken the physician's statements on faith.

Patients have access to more information. The most obvious new source of information is the Internet, and millions of patients have learned to do online research on their illnesses or complaints. And though much information on the Internet is bogus, much is both reliable and authoritative. Patients with sufficient education are usually perfectly capable of distinguishing between the good information and the bad. Then, too, newspapers, magazines, and television are providing more and more health news. Patients with particular interests will pick up on the new developments reported in the media and then turn to the Internet for additional information.

Patients have more money at stake. Health insurance bills are projected to continue to rise significantly in the years to come, still outpacing inflation. In an attempt to save money, employers and insurers have shifted some of these costs onto individual employees through higher premium sharing, copayments, and deductibles. Health insurance premiums rose 14 percent in 2003 and rose a total of 49 percent for family coverage between 2000 and 2003 (Kaiser Family Foundation and Health Research and Education Trust 2003). These costs added up: nearly one-quarter of insured families, for instance, spent $2,000 or more on their healthcare in a year. High out-of-pocket health costs contribute to medical bills being the second most frequently cited reason for bankruptcy in the nation as a whole. Among those polled in the study, about 80 percent were covered under some form of health insurance (Jacoby, Sullivan, and Warren 2001). When asked in a poll which healthcare issue currently facing them is the most important, 47 percent of consumers picked "affordability"—more than three times the number who chose "quality," which was second in importance at 13 percent (*Consortium Connection* 2003). Not surprisingly, consumers reason that if they are paying the bill, they want to know what they will receive for their money.

The consumerist trend—for good and ill—can be seen in one phenomenon that simply did not exist a decade ago. As the Food and Drug Administration (FDA) relaxed its restrictions on consumer-oriented pharmaceutical advertising, drug manufacturers began devoting more and more resources to direct-to-consumer (DTC) advertising. Between 1996 and 2001, for instance, DTC spending rose from $0.8 billion to $2.7 billion, an increase of more than threefold. Moreover, the ads were having an effect. According to a study by the Kaiser Family Foundation (2003), the proportion of the public saying they had seen or heard an ad for a prescription drug rose from 63 percent in 1997 to 85 percent in 2002. About one-third of adults said that they had discussed with their doctor a drug that they had seen advertised, and 44 percent of that group received a prescription for the medication in question. Thus, 13 percent of Americans "have received a specific prescription in response to seeing a drug ad" (Kaiser Family Foundation 2003, 5).

Both patients and physicians feel ambivalent about DTC advertising. Surveys by FDA researcher Kathryn J. Aikin (2003) found that more than half of patients agreed with the statements, "I like seeing advertisements for prescription drugs" and "Advertisements for prescription drugs help make me aware of new drugs." However, an even higher percentage agreed with the statements, "Advertisements for prescription drugs do not give enough information about the possible risks and negative effects of using the drug" and "Advertisements for prescription drugs make the drugs seem better than they really are." As for physicians, a significant minority (about 40 percent) felt that DTC advertising had beneficial effects on the patient-doctor relationship, largely because the ads facilitated "better discussion with patients" and because patients were "more aware of treatments." But some physicians felt they had to spend unnecessary time correcting patients' misperceptions about the drugs in question, and many felt that patients were poorly informed about topics such as who should and should not use the drug and what the possible risks and side-effects might be (Aikin 2003).

It is not surprising, of course, that physicians would agree to go along with reasonable patient requests, whether or not they are inspired by DTC advertising. In managed care plans, a prime directive is typically to maintain the patient base, and giving patients what they ask for is a way of keeping them happy. Every physician, moreover, is likely to feel pressed for time, and talking patients out of something they want is likely to take a lot more time than giving them what they want. Physicians thus often take the path of least resistance and get patients in and out more quickly. This may be one of many factors leading to unnecessary treatments such as the overprescribing of antibiotics. According to one study, 82 percent of physicians in general practice and 94 percent of infectious disease specialists agreed that antibiotic resistance is a major public health problem, and more than 80 percent cited patient demand as a major reason for antibiotic overprescribing (Metlay et al. 2002).[1] In addition, doctors know that patients must manage their own health; they are the ones who must actually get the prescription filled and take their medicine. Research confirms that patients are more likely to take a drug that they have requested than a drug with which they are unfamiliar (Handlin et al. 2003). "The data seem to suggest a positive association between advertising and compliance," says Nancy Ostrove, deputy director of the FDA's Division of Drug Marketing, Advertising, and Communications (*MediaDaily News* 2002).

THE NEW PARTNERSHIP

What seems to be emerging is a new model of healthcare, one in which patients are partners in their own care and in which providers are more tightly regulated, either by rules or by the availability of information. This may not be a bad thing, particularly because patients (especially those with chronic diseases) must take responsibility for much of their own care anyway. Healthcare providers are accepting this new mission. They use phrases such as, "Our mission is to help people manage their own health," or "We are helping people help themselves."

Trust, of course, is an essential element of this partnership. When patients mistrust their caregivers, they are much less effective partners. Building trust requires an awareness on both sides that there is a new relationship and that it requires mutual exchange of information. The watchword is not so much *caveat emptor*—buyer beware—as it is buyer be aware. "Ye shall know the truth," according to the Bible in John 8:32, "and the truth shall make you free." Truth—and trust—may also help produce better healthcare. The question is whether healthcare providers and organizations can understand the need for trust and the benefits it provides and whether they can build their capacity and their reputations around trust.

NOTE

1. Interestingly, only 36 percent and 22 percent of generalists and infectious disease specialists, respectively, admit to overprescribing antibiotics themselves.

REFERENCES

Aiken, L. H., S. P. Clarke, D. M. Sloane, J. Sochalski, and J. H. Silber. 2002. "Hospital Nurse Staffing and Patient Mortality, Nurse Burnout, and Job Dissatisfaction." *Journal of the American Medical Association* 288 (16): 1987–93.

Aikin, K. J. 2003. "The Impact of Direct-to-Consumer Prescription Drug Advertising on the Physician-Patient Relationship." Division of Drug Marketing, Advertising, and Communications, U.S. Food and Drug Administration, Sept. 22. [Online presentation; retrieved 10/7/03.] http://www.fda.gov/cder/ddmac/aikin/tsld001.htm.

Consortium Connection. 2003. "Understanding Market Expectations." *Consortium Connection* Winter: 4.

Goldstein, A. 2003. "For Patients' Rights, a Quiet Fadeaway." *Washington Post* Sept. 12, A4.

Handlin, A., J. B. Mosca, D. A. Forgione, and D. Pitta. 2003. "DTC Pharmaceutical Advertising: The Debate's Not Over." *Journal of Consumer Marketing* 20 (2/3): 227–38.

Jacoby, M. B., T. A. Sullivan, and E. Warren. 2001. "Rethinking the Debates over Health Care Financing: Evidence from the Bankruptcy Courts." *New York University Law Review* 2 (76): 377.

Kaiser Family Foundation. 2003. *Impact of Direct-to-Consumer Advertising on Prescription Drug Spending*, 5. [Online report; retrieved 11/18/04.] http://www.kff.org/rxdrugs/6084-index.cfm.

Kaiser Family Foundation and Health Educational and Research Trust. 2003. *Employer Health Benefits 2003 Annual Survey*. Chicago: Health Research and Educational Trust.

MediaDaily News. 2002. "Benefit to Public Health Lost in Debate over DTC Advertising." [Online article; retrieved 2/15/02.] www.mediapost.com.

Metlay, J. P., J. A. Shea, L. B. Crosette, and D. A. Asch. 2002. "Tensions in Antibiotic Prescribing: Pitting Social Concerns Against the Interests of Individual Patients." *Journal of General Internal Medicine* 17 (Feb.): 91.

Sacramento Bee. 2003. "California Governor Announces Regulations Governing Nurse-Patient Ratios." *Sacramento Bee* Sept. 30, D1.

PART II

Building Trust—And a Trusted Reputation

CHAPTER SIX

Thinking Differently

> No enterprise can exist for itself alone. It ministers to some great need; it performs some great service, not for itself, but for others; or failing therein, it ceases to be profitable and ceases to exist.
>
> —*Calvin Coolidge*

BY NOW I hope that you will agree with me about the dimensions of the trust crisis—the trust famine—in American healthcare. It is an ailment that needs treatment. Healthcare organizations are mistrusted not only by consumers and patients but also by key stakeholders, employees, and each other. Individual providers often enjoy high levels of trust, but that trust is in constant danger of being undermined. The media exacerbate the problem. Consumers clamor for a new level of involvement in their own care. Neither government regulation nor industry self-regulation has proved effective in restoring trust. If the problem is to be solved, it will be solved by healthcare leaders who understand it and take action to resolve it. It will be solved by individual professionals and managers who learn how to build trust in their practices, their units or services, and their organizations. It will be solved by people who understand what it takes to build a *reputation* for trust—a reputation so solid and durable that people simply take it for granted that the organization in question can be trusted. This in a nutshell is the "trust prescription for healthcare."

The chapters that follow will help you get started building the reputation needed to fill that prescription.

WHAT BUSINESS ARE YOU IN?

First, however, ask yourself what business you are in. Take note: this is not a simple question. Developing an answer to it can involve transforming your organization; it is also the starting point for understanding and implementing the trust prescription.

Hospitals, physicians' offices, managed care companies, pharmaceutical manufacturers, and many other kinds of organizations make up America's healthcare enterprise. Ask the chief executives and managers of all such organizations what business they are in, and they are likely to reply, "We are in healthcare." Some with a grander vision might respond, "We are in the business of saving lives." And, of course, both of these answers are true. But it is also true that *every company in the industry can respond the same way*. In other words, saying that you are in the healthcare business gives the people you are trying to reach—consumers, patients, professionals, investors, donors, and so on—no way to distinguish your organization from every other similar organization, including your competition.

So let us look from a different angle at this question of what business you are in. To help gain perspective, we will search out some lessons from other industries. My point in looking for lessons elsewhere is emphatically *not* that healthcare is "just a business like any other." Healthcare is indeed a business, but it is an unusual one. It routinely deals with life-and-death issues. The people it serves are not usually called customers; they are called patients. Many of its key employees think of themselves as clinicians and professionals, not businesspeople. ("Lawyers and prostitutes have clients and customers," read an angry button worn by surgeons who were pushed by a managed care company to attend a customer service seminar. "Doctors have *patients*.") A large fraction of the sector operates on a not-for-profit basis, both in theory (that is, the way the organizations are set up) and in fact (they do not make money). To say that healthcare is a business like any other is to ignore what makes the healthcare enterprise unique.

Still, bear with me while we take a side jaunt into the world of business as practiced by other industries. It is worth doing, because we all need some innovative thinking. Healthcare is facing a crisis right now, and the leaders of the healthcare sector could benefit from new ideas about how to address it.

WHAT IS A COMPANY SELLING?

To begin, consider the automobile industry. Here is a quick, fairly simple short-answer test. Can you identify the qualities that each car brand wants to be identified with?

1. BMW	a. Adventure and excitement
2. Jeep	b. Value and reliability
3. Mercedes	c. Safety
4. Toyota	d. High performance
5. Volvo	e. Solid engineering

This is simple enough that you hardly need the answers (1d, 2a, 3e, 4b, 5c). But that is partly the point. Auto companies typically do not just market cars; they market something special about those cars. They position themselves in the marketplace, and in the mind of the potential customer, as offering something unique. They repeat the message in every possible way. But note an important point about this positioning: in the best cases—the most successful companies—it is not simply a marketing ploy that goes into the company's advertising. Rather, the company builds its entire operation around what makes it unique. Toyota's cars really *are* exceptionally reliable, in part because of the company's pioneering approach to manufacturing quality and continuous improvement.

Mercedes cars really *are* well-engineered; engineers occupy pride of place within the organization.

Consider Volvo, which is known worldwide for safety. Volvo makes very safe cars, but so do many other manufacturers. No matter; ask a car buyer what the safest car is, and the chances are good that he or she will say a Volvo. That is because everything Volvo does is geared toward creating and communicating a single message. Its design engineers are obsessed with safety and spend long hours designing cars that will protect their occupants in case of a crash. (It is even said that Volvo's engineers were late to add built-in cupholders, because they considered drinking coffee while driving an unsafe practice.) The company's ads carry safety-related slogans ("Volvo—for life"). Its brochures are printed on thick, durable paper and emphasize Volvo's commitment to safety. The Volvo promise is captured in a quote from its founders: "The guiding principle behind everything we do at Volvo is and must remain safety." It is represented by the first sentence that appears on the "Why Volvo" page of the company's web site: "For over 75 years, the design of every Volvo has been guided by our concern for the safety and well-being of people" (Volvocars.com 2004).

Look also at what Volvo does not do. It does not produce inexpensive cars aimed at 22-year-olds. It does not emphasize its cars' gas mileage, styling, luxury, or performance; if it mentions these features at all, they come well behind safety. Nor does Volvo do things like sponsor wrestling tournaments or NASCAR races; instead, it makes a large grant every year to the journal *Spine* for the best research article. Everything it does is relevant to the brand's positioning. In a very real sense, Volvo is not in the car business; it is in the safety business.

Now let us broaden our horizons and look at other industries. Here is another test, a little bit tougher than the first. Can you identify what each company is selling, along with its products or services?

1. Amazon.com	A. Youth
2. Bic	B. Meeting place
3. Disney	C. Disposability

4. Fannie Mae	D. Distribution
5. Nike	E. Magic
6. Starbucks	F. Heroism
7. Revlon	G. Service
8. Woolite	H. Gentleness
9. Nordstrom	I. American dream
10. Pepsi	J. Hope

Charles Revson, founder of Revlon, is said to have put the matter succinctly: "In the factory we make cosmetics; in the store we sell hope" (Knowles 2003). Buy the right lipstick, runs the Revlon message, and you too will be young, attractive, and desirable. Though it is easy to dismiss Revson's approach (or Pepsi's youth-oriented marketing) as cynical, nearly every leading company offers the buyer something other than just a product or service. Fannie Mae, a participant in the secondary mortgage market, never mentions home loans *per se*; it says, "Our business is the American dream" (fanniemae.com 2004). Nike rarely mentions shoes; its ads show heroic athletes just doing it. Woolite does not sell laundry soap, which is a means to an end; it sells the end itself, namely the gentleness of the fabrics that are washed with Woolite.

Whole business models are built around the idea that a company's real business can be quite different from what it seems to be. Starbucks founder Howard Schultz has always been clear that his company is not in the coffee business; it is in the business of providing people a place to meet and talk. Bic has defined its business not as pens—its first product—but as disposability, which allowed it to migrate easily to disposable razors and lighters. Amazon founder Jeff Bezos always knew that his company was not a glorified bookstore; it was a distribution system—which meant it could (and does) sell dozens of different retail products. Imagine for a moment that Nordstrom decided to open a travel agency or a hotel. Your immediate assumption would be that the new business would be characterized by topflight service, because that—not just clothing—is what you always associate with Nordstrom.

Like Volvo, a successful company positions itself around its "real" business and reinforces the message in dozens of different ways. Take Disney. Is this company in the movie business, the theme park business, the entertainment business? The answer "all of the above" wins only partial credit, because Disney is first and foremost in the magic business. When you enter a Disney facility—the Magic Kingdom—the first thing you see are signs using the word magic. You will find the word magic repeated at multiple points at which the customer has contact with Disney, from signage to staff greetings to souvenirs. Disney takes the brand promise of magic and delivers it consistently, across all of the company's product lines and channels of distribution, and over a sustained period of time. While staying at a Disney-owned hotel, I oberseved the following strategy employed on an internal advertising channel:

- We are invited to "imagine the magic" of our next Disney vacation.
- Disney Cruise Line offers "a voyage into uncharted magic"; Disney's Castaway Key Island is "the most magical island ever discovered."
- Disney Paris asks us to "come and live the magic," Tokyo Disney to "come experience the magic."
- Disney's Vero Beach offers us "waves of magic," Disney's time share a chance to "own a piece of the magic."

Plenty of companies are in those other businesses that Disney participates in—theme parks, movies, entertainment, cruises—but not one other than Disney is in the magic business.

THE THINGS THAT MATTER MOST

These positioning tactics reflect some fundamental truths about operating in a marketplace—any marketplace.

The Best Quality Does Not Automatically Win Market Leadership

Knowledgeable information technology professionals know that Microsoft is not the only company to offer a quality operating system for personal computers. Marketing experts understand that Coca-Cola does not always win taste tests. Those whose trade is home appliances know that Maytag, the dependability company, is not the only company to make dependable appliances. But it does not matter: these companies are market leaders because they understand that quality alone is not sufficient to carve out a distinctive position in the minds of consumers.

Do not misinterpret the importance of positioning to mean that quality is irrelevant. Quality matters a great deal. Volvo could never set itself up in the safety business unless its cars were very safe indeed. Disney could not offer magic unless it really was capable of offering its customers exceptional entertainment experiences. But in most industries these days, quality is no more than a ticket to entry, just as we saw in earlier chapters that competence is no more than a ticket to entry into healthcare. Research shows very clearly that most major brands have parity: consumers do not see much difference between the products and services that they offer, *except on the basis of the intangibles that the company adds to the brand.* Which of us, when planning a family vacation, wants to sit down and laboriously compare the rides, attractions, prices, and facilities that are offered by Disney, Universal, Six Flags, or other competitors? So we do not—we buy the magic. Disney in effect has put itself into a different category. Which of us, when buying a car, wants to compare government crash tests for a dozen brands? If safety is our primary concern, we want to buy a safe car with the highest ratings, which Volvo repeatedly receives, but we also want to feel that the whole company is dedicated to safety. Volvo can be trusted to make a safe car. So we buy a Volvo.

Perception Is Reality—and Emotion Trumps Reason

Aristotle recognized that people make decisions with their emotions as well as their reason, with their hearts as well as their heads. Marketers, of course, know this truth very well, which is why advertising and other marketing techniques conjure up emotional responses. The power of these emotional responses cannot be overstated. People buy Tide rather than some other laundry detergent because their mothers did and because they feel good about the association. They buy Nike sneakers rather than a cheaper (but equally good) competitor's pair because they yearn to be like the athletes in the ads.

There is no more dramatic example of the power of emotion than Coca-Cola, perhaps the preeminent branded product in today's global economy. Coke is little more than brown-colored, carbonated sugar water with a little flavoring. People like its taste, but they also like the taste of many of its competitors (Coke has regularly lost blind taste tests) (Pendergrast 2000). But never mind how mundane a product it may be: it has a billion daily drinkers worldwide and adds about a million new drinkers every day.

Remember what happened when the company tried to change the formula and introduce "New Coke"? The public went crazy. There were pickets at Coca-Cola's Atlanta headquarters. There were lawsuits to have the original formula released. There were even a couple of hunger strikes. Roberto Goizueta, CEO at the time and arguably the greatest brand builder of the twentieth century, was puzzled; he had been obsessed with beating Pepsi in blind taste tests (the "Pepsi challenge"), and New Coke performed better than Classic Coke on these tests. What he failed to realize is that it was never about the taste of Coke. The taste may be what Coke advertises, but it is not what Coke sells. It sells family, fun, and friendships; it sells good times, nostalgia, and patriotism. The closest description of what it sells might be, "America in a bottle." All of these concepts conjure up strong emotions. Monkeying with the formula for Coke was somehow like monkeying with the formula for America. In a way, Coca-Cola did not know its own power.

Recognize the Importance of Being Distinctive

Notice, however, how Coca-Cola hedges its bets. Other soft drink companies can advertise themselves as part of Americana, too. But their drinks are not Coke—and the reason is that only Coke has that top-secret formula known as Merchandise 7X. The company likes to remind us that the formula is more carefully guarded than the formula for the hydrogen bomb. (You can probably find the bomb recipe on the Internet, but not the Coke recipe.) Everything else about Coke's presentation to the consumer reinforces the notion of distinctiveness: the Spenserian script logo, the ubiquitous red color, even the distinctive contour bottle, which regularly makes an appearance in the supermarket even though it has long since been supplanted by cans and conventional two-liter plastic bottles as the containers of choice.

So it is with the other companies we have mentioned. By now, a car company that chose to emphasize safety above all else would be dismissed as a Volvo wannabe. Volvo owns safety, and no one can easily emulate it. Anybody can build a theme park, but only Disney can build a magical one populated by the famous Disney characters and built around the famous Disney stories. Disney owns magic. These and many other companies stand for something in the mind of the marketplace. They occupy a market position that they have carved out, fortified, and learned to defend against all comers, because it is unique.

The German poet Goethe said, "The things that matter most should never be at the mercy of the things that matter least." Coke, Disney, and Volvo know this and are careful to organize their businesses so that what matters most—their position in the marketplace—dominates every facet of their operations, day in and day out.

INTRODUCING: THE POWER BRAND

What is created through this attention to positioning—to the business that these companies are really in—is something that might be called a *power brand.* Everybody knows about brands and branding. Companies create brands. Marketers study them; they speak in terms of "brand architecture" and "brand elasticity." Anybody who watches TV advertising knows about the ongoing brand wars (a classic of a few years ago was Miller Lite versus Bud Light). But power brands are a breed apart. A power brand is something consumers are willing to pay more for, travel farther for, wait longer for. A power brand dominates its marketplace. Disney, Coke, and Volvo are all power brands. So is Harley-Davidson motorcycles—what other brand do you know that people tattoo on their bodies? Power brands attract new customers more easily than others do and convert them more easily into long-term, loyal "brand demanders." They enjoy "share of mind" in the marketplace, and are able to capture and retain "share of heart." The products or services they offer are viewed by consumers not only as excellent but as distinctive.

The magic of a power brand is that it creates a halo effect over an entire organization. A company with a power brand attracts the best and brightest employees; who would not want to work for a name that is known and trusted by everyone? It serves as a protective firewall in the face of adversity. A power brand means something, and in the chapters that follow we will see how to create one.

THE LESSONS FOR HEALTHCARE

First, let us return to the healthcare business. It was Picasso who said, "Good artists copy, but great artists steal." Healthcare leaders may want to begin stealing from other industries. The lessons just covered have some interesting implications.

There Are Very Few Power Brands in Healthcare

Those power brands that exist in healthcare can practically be counted on the fingers of one hand. The Mayo Clinic is certainly a power brand. Johnson & Johnson is another. But who else? Perhaps we could argue about the Cleveland Clinic or the Massachusetts General Hospital, Blue Cross–Blue Shield, or Kaiser Permanente. But soon we would be stretching the concept to its breaking point. The fact is, with only a few exceptions, there are no names in healthcare that consumers automatically assume are head and shoulders above the rest because they occupy a distinctive space in the marketplace. There are ever so few that consumers will pay more for, travel farther for, and wait longer for.

Few companies in healthcare even understand what goes into creating a power brand. They advertise their quality, as if quality were more than merely a ticket to enter the marketplace. Hospitals say they are accredited and that their physicians are board certified. Managed care plans advertise that you can choose your own doctor. Pharmaceutical companies tell us that their pills will cure our ills. But is there a single statement here that is unique or distinctive or that the hospital or the managed care plan or the pharmaceutical company down the street cannot say with equal conviction? Is there anything at all that taps into people's emotional need to patronize a company they believe in and trust? I fear that the answer is no.

To put the matter only a little differently, few healthcare organizations have any idea of what business they might really be in. They are stuck. They believe that they occupy this or that niche in the healthcare industry, and they never think of what they might have to offer the world that would set them apart from the pack. Yet as we have seen, that is precisely what puts great companies in a different category from run-of-the-mill ones: they sell something else, something that transcends mere products and services and that no one else can copy.

A tale is told of the two shoe salesmen many years ago who arrived in an underdeveloped tropical country. One observed that no one in the country wore shoes and promptly left for home, figuring there was no market. The other wired back to headquarters, "Huge opportunity here—send more salespeople." So it is with healthcare: the absence of power brands does not mean that these fundamental lessons in marketing, such as knowing what business you are really in, are not applicable. Rather it means that this is wide-open territory and that there is an immense opportunity here for organizations that want to learn those lessons.

What is more, there is a particular opportunity for organizations that want to respond to the crisis that is the subject of this book: the trust crisis. Imagine for a moment what it might be like if *you* were thinking differently, if your practice or service or organization saw itself not only in the healthcare business but in the trust business. Imagine that you were the one player that consumers immediately trusted, with their hearts as well as their heads, because your trustworthiness was what distinguished you from everybody else. Imagine that you owned a power brand built around trust.

Read on, and you will learn how to create one.

REFERENCES

Fanniemae.com. 2004. Home page. [Online information; retrieved 11/22/04.] http://www.fanniemae.com/index.jhtml.

Knowles, E. 2003. "Revson, Charles." In *The Oxford Dictionary of Modern Quotations, Second Edition,* 273. New York: Oxford University Press.

Pendergrast, M. 2000. *For God, Country and Coca Cola: The Definitive History of the Great American Soft Drink and the Company that Makes It,* 312, 333, 376. New York: Basic Books.

Volvocars.com. 2004. "Why Volvo." [Online information; retrieved 11/22/04.] http://www.volvocars.us/_Tier2/WhyVolvo/.

CHAPTER SEVEN

Understanding Branding

A good organization produces excellent programs, products, and services.

A great one—a power brand—is *trusted* to consistently deliver excellent programs, products, and services that are *perceived* by consumers to be both *relevant* and *distinctive.*

THIS CHAPTER—INDEED, the rest of this book—is about building a power brand based on trust. The words shown in italics above are important in this journey, and I will return to each one. In preparation, and in keeping with the previous chapter's excursion into other businesses, I explain why I unabashedly use the language and concepts of brands and branding in a field such as healthcare, which has traditionally avoided such notions.

Many people in healthcare work in the field precisely because they did not want to go into business. They are uncomfortable with words such as *customers* and *marketing*. Branding—which smacks of Madison Avenue and hucksterism—may be one of the least popular concepts among healthcare professionals. "We will do good work," many are inclined to think, "and create an excellent organization. We will devote our resources to serving patients, not to advertising. People will find us because of our sterling reputation."

Unfortunately, to think this way is to misunderstand the nature of a brand and to miss out on a chance to serve more patients even more effectively. Three points are critical.

First, every organization already has a brand. The brand may be explicit or implicit, widely publicized or not. It may be powerful or weak, cultivated or ignored. *Brand* is just shorthand for the position that the organization occupies in the mind of the marketplace. Unless a company or practice is completely unknown—not, presumably, what anybody wishes for—it is always perceived as good, bad, or indifferent (or some combination thereof) by those whom it is attempting to serve. Surely you have heard word-of-mouth evidence of this fact: "The radiology unit at Memorial Hospital is the best in the city," or "Nobody would be on that health plan if they had a choice." Your brand already exists, as a matter of course. What you do with it is up to you.

Second, branding is simply a way of locating yourself in the marketplace so that you are what you choose to be—and so that that the marketplace thinks of you that way. Marketers call this positioning, and it is a critical component of any successful organization's fundamental strategy. Far from being limited to advertising, publicity, or any other single tool, positioning is essentially a process of organizational development. It means identifying the organization's mission, vision, and values. It means establishing a reputation—a position—in the market. Companies with power brands ensure that everything the organization does is relevant to that reputation. Remember the lessons of the previous chapter: Volvo does not make inexpensive cars for 22-year-olds, nor does it sponsor NASCAR races. Only when its position is established organizationally does the company take its message to the marketplace through advertising and the other techniques of marketing.

Third, establishing a trusted brand is one of the most effective ways of appealing to the people you want to serve. As we have seen, a power brand sets you apart. It attracts customers, professionals, employees, donors or investors, and business partners. It encourages compliance, referrals, and loyalty. It enables an organization to pursue its mission while realizing a healthy margin. It serves as a protective firewall in the face of adversity. With a power brand, when something goes amiss, a person is likely to give it a second chance, or better yet, the benefit of the doubt. To ignore the power of a trusted brand is to ignore one of the most potent tools available for building an effective, durable organization.

Let us establish a common language and common ground by considering some of the basics of branding. Then I will outline a comprehensive, market-tested model for developing and implementing a power brand.

BRAND ARCHITECTURE

The executives of such companies as Procter & Gamble (P&G) and Johnson & Johnson have to concern themselves with *brand architecture*, meaning the positioning of a wide range of products in diverse marketplaces. Tide, Cheer, and Era, for example, are all manufactured by P&G; each is designed to appeal to a slightly different segment of P&G's target markets. Procter & Gamble is known as a "house of brands" because it has so many different branded products, each with its own name and each only loosely identified with the parent company. By contrast, organizations such as General Electric (GE) and Harvard University are examples of what is known as a "branded house." The parent's name appears prominently in the name of nearly every subsidiary (GE Medical System, Harvard School of Public Health, GE Global Research). The parent is very much perceived in the marketplace as an organization, not simply a loose collection of products or services.

Only a few healthcare executives must concern themselves with a large array of brands, but the issues of brand architecture may still be relevant to many. If you are the CEO of a large hospital, do you focus your efforts on the hospital's overall brand, or do you focus instead on branding your birthing center, your cardiology service, or your new sports medicine unit? If you run an insurance company, how much should you invest in promoting the company's brand as opposed to the subbrands of the various insurance programs you offer? If you are a physician in a group practice, do you want the practice's name to be uppermost in your patients' minds, or do you want them to think of your name first?

Executives and professionals sometimes fail to think through such questions and, as a result, fall into a couple of potential traps. They may invest halfheartedly in both the parent brand and the subbrands, without devoting the effort needed to make either one stand out in the marketplace. Worse, they may find that the parent brand and one or more subbrands occupy conflicting positions in the marketplace. Such a problem has cropped up repeatedly in the airline business whenever a major airline attempts to establish a no-frills, low-cost subsidiary service to compete with Southwest Airlines. The parent typically does not want travelers to forget that the new subsidiary is backed by an established airline, but why, then, should travelers believe that the subsidiary will be any different from the high-cost, full-service airline that they are used to?

The fundamental question raised by brand architecture, of course, is where you want the brand equity to lie. That will be a question to keep in mind as we explore the other basics of branding.

POSITIONING: THE BRAND PROMISE

Positioning—locating your products, services, programs, or organization in the minds of consumers—is your promise to the people you want to serve. It tells them the reasons for your brand's existence. It also tells them how and why you are different from everybody else. A position or *brand promise* is a landscape of your own choosing: with it, you become the architect of your own destiny. If a brand is a promise that leads to a preference in the marketplace, then your positioning statement is that promise.

What should your positioning—your brand promise—be? Alas, that is not a question that allows a quick answer. It entails spending a considerable amount of effort ascertaining exactly what you want your organization to be and then developing a branding

Positioning Promises

Analyze a company's positioning promise, and you typically find three key elements: a target market, a category or frame of reference, and a key benefit or point of difference. Note how the following examples contain each one:

- *To Senior Plan subscribers, SeniorChoice is the brand of Medicare health plan that provides low-cost benefits to more seniors in western New York than any other health plan.*
- *When seeking good health, you can trust the Baptist family to minister to your body, mind, and spirit with exceptional care and compassion. (Baptist Health System)*

strategy around that mission and vision. However, although there are no quick answers, there are some criteria that any positioning statement must meet.

First, it must offer a benefit. Volvo promises safety. Wal-Mart promises everyday low prices. Less astute organizations simply tout themselves as "the best" or some other such phrase, leaving consumers to wonder what that might mean to them. Of course, a benefit can be—and often is—emotional as well as rational. Pepsi does not just say it will quench your thirst; it promises that you will feel young, a part of the Pepsi Generation.

Second, the benefit must be relevant to the people it is aimed at. Disney promises magic at every opportunity, because the consumers it wants to attract—parents of young children—know that "magic" will appeal to their kids. Johnson & Johnson's baby shampoo carries its benefit right in its name: No More Tears. Every parent knows why that is valuable.

Third, the promise must be credible. It must fit with the organization. Tyco, site of one of the major corporate scandals that occurred recently, could not suddenly announce itself as "the company you can trust." ExxonMobil could not position itself as the company that protects your environment even now, years after the disaster caused by the *Exxon Valdez*. Nordstrom can and does

Positioning Promise Worksheet

Use this worksheet to develop your own positioning promise.

To ____

[Target market]

Brand X is the

(only)____

[Frame of reference]

that____

____

[Key benefit or statement of need fulfillment]

because____

____.

[Relevant support]

promise service of legendary quality because the organization is built around providing that kind of service.

Fourth, the promise must be scalable. It must be able to cover the entirety of whatever is being branded. Revlon cosmetics promise hope—and hope can be associated with any of its products that make a woman feel more attractive. Fannie Mae is able to promise the American dream of home ownership only because its primary business is mortgage loans. If it were also to pursue a major business in, say, currency trading, the promise would be meaningless.

Fifth, the promise must be enduring. A positioning promise, a brand identity, is something that never—or very rarely—changes. This attribute is more important than any particular characteristic of the brand itself. We know instantly what Rolls-Royce and Wal-Mart stand for, not because their brand promises resemble each other but because the two brands have each stood for the same thing for so long. By contrast, ask yourself what Pontiac or even Sears stands for. Sears's advertising campaigns at one time promised us "the softer side of Sears," even while simultaneously promoting Craftsman chain saws.

Assessing a Positioning Statement

Not every positioning statement is effective. At a minimum, it must pass the following screens:

- Is it consistent? Does it fit with the organization?
- Is it credible and relevant? Will consumers believe it—and will it matter to them?
- Is it internally adoptable? Professionals and staff must be prepared to buy in.
- Is it scalable across the entire enterprise?
- Is it distinctive? A valid position is one that competitors cannot easily emulate.
- Is it sustainable and durable? It must be "evergreen."
- Is it meaningful, memorable, epic? The best positioning statements are ambitious.
- Is it concise?
- Is it realistic? If you cannot pull it off, do not even try.

Finally, the promise must be distinctive, and hence different from what the competition is promising. After all, it is the competition and not the customer that determines market share and profitability, because the options in the market go a long way in determining where any entity fits. Specifically, competition has a predominant influence on pricing and the amount of business any one entity receives. Yet many companies and organizations seem to ignore the need to differentiate themselves, or at least are unsuccessful in doing so. In healthcare, nearly every organization has access to the same medicines, the same equipment, the same pool of professionals and staff. What makes one organization different from another?

CLIMBING UP THE BRAND HIERARCHY

Branding is a dynamic process. It is a process by which a brand evolves or migrates, gaining value along the way. The mental real

Figure 7.1. Laddering Up the Brand

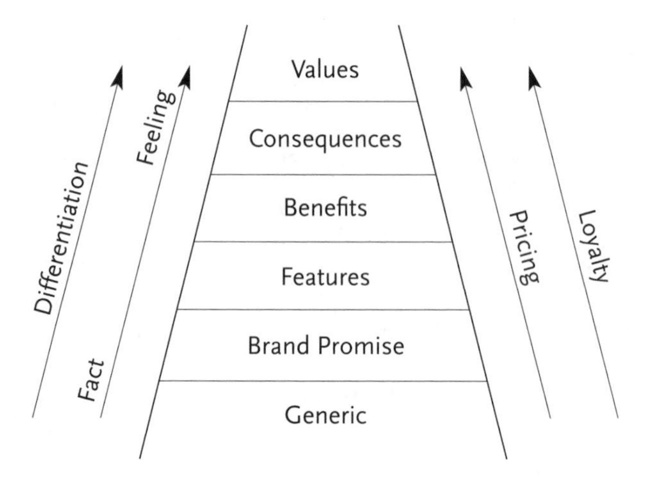

Source: © 2005, David A. Shore

estate that a brand can occupy is usually progressive. Of course, the internal process of building a brand is quite precise, and a future power brand will have the top rung of the ladder in mind strategically during its design. This process will be discussed in Chapter 11. However, a brand should expect to progress through the rungs of the brand equity ladder from the perspective of the market, as a process of evolution (see Figure 7.1).

The lowest rung on the branding ladder is the unattended or meaningless brand, the one that is not cultivated or differentiated from the competition. Generic and commodity products never get beyond this level. If you buy a bag of rock salt to melt the ice on your walk, you probably do not know and do not care about the manufacturer. If you buy a dozen peaches at the supermarket, you do not know and do not care about who grew them or who distributed them. Many brands never move beyond this level; they remain undifferentiated and undistinguished.

The next rung is a brand that promises something, which is the entry ticket to the higher rungs. The question, of course, is what the brand promises and whether the consumer ultimately receives the benefit of that promise. The lowest level of promise focuses on the product's or service's *features*. This truck has four-wheel drive and a V-8 engine. This insurance policy offers nationwide coverage. This computer works at blazing speed. Here, too, many brands get stuck: they leave us wondering why we should care about these features when we really need to know what the brand will do for us. So the next level of promise focuses on *benefits* to the consumer. Marketers put it like this: Don't tell me about your grass seed, tell me about my lawn. All I really want to know about the grass seed is whether my lawn will be healthy and as green as my neighbor's.

The features-to-benefits migration is a subject for Marketing 101: no company that takes its brand seriously ignores the importance of showing the benefits to the buyer. That is why you see active young couples enjoying the wilderness in their Jeeps and why insurance companies tout the peace of mind that they offer. The makers of Pampers and Huggies do not promote their product's absorbency capacities; they promote the benefits of a dry baby. "We don't sell software," reads the ad for one software company's products, "we sell advantage."

The upper rungs of the brand hierarchy, however, are reserved for the owners of power brands. For the fact is, a kind of transformation occurs when a brand migrates from features and benefits to consequences and values.

Why should this be? "It is not enough to appeal to reason and logic," wrote Aristotle; "we must also appeal to the emotions." Where the lower rungs involve reason and logic—here are the facts, here are the benefits you can expect—the upper rungs involve emotions. They capitalize on the long-term consequences of a purchase and the values that the purchaser wants to realize. Moving up to the top rungs of the brand ladder entails creating an emotional bond with the consumer that is far stronger than any purely rational attachment can ever be.

A real-world example may clarify the point. The key feature of Johnson & Johnson's baby shampoo is its mildness; the key benefit is contained in the name No More Tears. But it is the longer-term, emotion-based connection that matters here. "Tearless" shampoos create a better bath experience for parent and baby alike. The parent feels less like an ogre for shampooing the child and making her cry and more like a good parent, the kind of parent he wants to be. Johnson & Johnson reinforces this connection in its ads, in its promotional materials, and in its marketing strategy. In effect it sells the parent-infant bond, the kindness and gentleness that parents associate with taking care of babies, and the care that parents want to think they can offer their offspring. This is a powerful connection. It leaves parents who settle for some other shampoo—or some other whole line of baby products—wondering if they are doing the best thing possible for their children.

The rungs of the branding ladder are not mutually exclusive. Rather, they are iterative; you have to include the lower rungs as you move toward the higher ones. Branding begins with the facts of a product or service, moves on to the benefits it provides to the consumer, and (in the best circumstances) eventually migrates toward a long-term, emotional connection. A brand based on that emotional connection has meaning in a person's life; it turns the buyer from a *soft target,* meaning someone who can easily be swayed by a competitor's pitch, to a *hard target,* someone who remains loyal to the brand in question. Moving up the ladder entails moving from

- facts → feelings
- mind share → heart share
- undifferentiated → differentiated
- required → desired
- softer targets → harder targets
- merchandising → image advertising
- commodity → uniqueness

In effect, you begin to own some mental real estate in the marketplace; you build a reputation and provide people with reasons to believe in it. You move from an ordinary brand to a power brand, a brand in which people perceive quality and for which they are willing to pay more because they trust it.

THE SITUATION IN HEALTHCARE

Some of the companies that supply products to the healthcare industry—pharmaceutical manufacturers, makers of personal care products, medical equipment companies, and so on—are themselves power brands. The chief marketers at Pfizer, Johnson & Johnson, and GE Medical Systems do not need instruction in marketing. But how different the situation is when it comes to hospitals, nursing homes, medical practices, HMOs, and all the many other organizations and services that make up the direct care enterprise. We noted earlier that there are only a couple of power brands, such as the Mayo Clinic, in this part of the industry. The sad fact is, there are only a few brands that cultivate their status with strategic planning by a brand management committee, a necessity for power brands and aspiring brands.

The result is that most of the healthcare industry is at the commodity level of the brand hierarchy. Consumers cannot tell one provider from another. They make their choices on the basis of convenience, inertia, or a recommendation from a friend. Without branding, healthcare becomes a retail industry, and in retail, as in residential real estate, the three most important factors are location, location, and location. Thus, a hospital's or nursing home's success too often depends on where it happens to be. An HMO's success depends on which employers it can convince to carry it rather than on an active choice by consumers.

This commodity strategy worked tolerably well as long as demand for healthcare outstripped supply and as long as consumers went along with whatever their physician or employer recommended. Today's environment, of course, is quite different. No longer is there room in the marketplace for all of the institutions and organizations that once populated it. (Witness the closing of community hospitals in many areas of the country.) Customers—patients—are no longer necessarily willing to accept whatever their doctor recommends. They now have access through the Internet to all sorts of information about competing healthcare facilities, and they are voting with their feet. They will head for facilities and organizations that they believe stand for something, that occupy a position in their minds. They will head for facilities and organizations that develop a meaningful brand—a power brand.

Developing such a brand entails a journey into the heart of your organization. It involves following a series of sequential steps. Again, this is not a journey to be undertaken lightly. Each step requires a serious commitment of resources, including the time of senior management. Branding is not just marketing. It is the position adopted by the organization, and positioning in this sense requires attention from everybody. The worst possible thing you can do is stake out a positioning territory and then fail to be what you say you are. But if you are willing to make the commitment, the following chapters will show you how to figure out what you want to promise and how to create an organization that makes good on its promises.

CHAPTER EIGHT

Raison d'Être: Mission, Vision, and Values

Dream no small dreams, for they
have no power to move the heart.

—*Goethe*

ORGANIZATIONS REGULARLY ASK themselves the wrong questions: How can we do it better? How can we do it cheaper? How can we do it faster? These are all questions that may make sense once you know where you are going. But a better question to ask first is, Why do we do what we do at all? What is our *raison d'être*, our reason for being, the justification for our existence? This question gets at the heart of building a brand, because a brand that does not stand for something is hardly a brand at all. Before you can gain market share, before you can increase market penetration, before you can increase profitability and margin, before you should launch new products and services, you must make it clear, both internally and externally, what your organization is and what your brand stands for.

This is the beginning of the journey, phase one in the sequence of steps in building a power brand. At this point we are concerned with articulating a dream, not with building a plan; the planning will follow. The challenge here is to provide a framework for creating a deeper understanding among all key stakeholders of why your organization or enterprise exists. This is central to building a strong reputation and the increased brand equity that follows.

Determining your *raison d'être* begins with the organizational trinity of mission, vision, and values (MV^2). The trinity provides a three-pointed anchor for your brand, providing guidance and direction. Without defining and clarifying MV^2, alignment across divisions, departments, or staff groups and within product lines is nearly impossible. At the same time, aligning MV^2 enables brand strategy to successfully move on to brand development (phase two). Mission, vision, and values are the antecedents of brand development.

MV^2 itself is an organization's moral compass. It answers several questions, including the following:

- Why does your organization exist?
- What is the essence of its brand?
- What are its core beliefs, its philosophy of service?
- What does it do best, and how does that relate to what its target markets need?
- How can the brand really make a difference in the lives of its customers and in society?
- Where would you like the organization to be 3, 5, 10, or even 20 years from now?

These are no small questions. Answering them requires a voyage into the heart of the organization, not to mention a good deal of soul searching on the part of those responsible for it. Nor can C-level executives (CEO, COO, CIO, CNO, etc.) delegate this responsibility. If they do not get involved in the development of mission, vision, and values, nobody will take the exercise seriously.

Because MV^2 is at the heart of this phase, it is worth understanding some basics of what it should involve.

- This is a time for thinking big. No one gets excited about small dreams. People want grand ambitions, lofty goals, the highest standards. Be epic!
- The focus here is on the organization, not the brand. But strategic branding goals and objectives will be derived from MV^2, so whatever is created in this process must be owned by the organization. It will be the foundation for what comes later.

- MV^2 should inspire your employees. The ability to influence the larger society is based principally on an organization's ability to influence its own employees and other stakeholders. Your employees want to be loyal and committed. Give them a reason to be.
- MV^2 is primarily for internal consumption. It is inbound rather than outbound; it is for internal stakeholders such as employees, the board, and key business partners. Done right, it provides these stakeholders with a shared focus and direction and serves as the foundation of the organization's future growth and development. Once the core principles and beliefs are established, they should be widely circulated and regularly discussed throughout the organization to promote a common understanding and acceptance.

Oliver Wendell Holmes once said, "What lies behind us and what lies before us are tiny matters compared with what lies within us." If you want to make trust central to your brand—if you want to be known for trust—then this is where it begins: you must create a *raison d'être* in which trust is an essential component.

MISSION

An organization's *mission* is a written statement that is the focal point for all of its activities. Everything the organization does either supports and adds value to the mission or fails to support and add value to the mission. The mission statement is a declaration of the organization's ultimate purpose, a pronouncement of why the brand, and the organization itself, exist. The mission of the mission statement, so to speak, is to communicate that purpose to stakeholders and make it possible for them to believe in what it says. If employees and other stakeholders do not understand the noble purpose of the organization, how can they effectively support it?

Mission statements, to be sure, have a mixed reputation. They are often thought of as grandiose pronouncements destined for a dusty piece of parchment posted on the wall. In a poll reported in *Business Week*, 70 percent of American workers said that their organization had a mission statement, but only 41 percent had any idea what it was (Oleck 1998). In another poll, 48 percent of the 1,105 workers surveyed reported that mission statements were used rarely or sometimes to guide their actions (MeaningfulWorkplace.com 2000). Even at the executive level, it is common to hear the refrain, "No margin, no mission," as if "mission" was something that could safely be put aside until the company had gone about its real business of earning a profit. "Mission" is seen as soft when compared to the hard benchmarks of revenues, expenses, and earnings.

But the checkered career of mission statements should not discourage a company from doing it right. The point, after all, is not simply to have a mission statement but to actually have a *mission*. Establishing a mission that people can buy into brings clarity and commitment, without which you will never be able to deliver on your brand promise. Indeed, it is probably safer to say "No mission, no margin," than the converse.

The Process

There are (at least) two wrong ways to go about writing a mission statement, and there is one right way, which, unfortunately, is somewhat more difficult. Wrong Way No. 1 is to contract the work out. Perhaps the CEO decides that the organization needs a new mission statement and asks someone in corporate communications (or, worse, a consultant) to draft one for the chief's approval. The process is quick, it is easy, and it is utterly fruitless; such a mission statement is guaranteed to be vapid. And because no one in the organization has been involved in writing it, why would anyone buy into it?

Wrong Way No. 2—more common, but not much more effective—is to gather a team of senior executives, take them to a day-long offsite retreat, and ask them to come up with a statement. The problem here is not so much in sins of commission, as the procedure may indeed be a useful part of the overall process, but in sins of omission. There has been no preparation. There has been no attempt to involve anyone outside the limited circle of top executives. People are supposed to come up with a mission statement literally out of thin air. This, too, is a recipe for meaningless verbiage.

The right way is longer and more costly but ultimately more meaningful and more effective. It begins with brainstorming and dialog. Get people throughout the organization talking about what the organization's mission is. If there is a mission statement already in place, ask people to critique it. If practical, consider asking every employee to write a personal mission statement reflecting what he or she would like the organization to be. Consult board members and trusted outsiders. If trust is to be a central part of the mission, as I would hope, ask people what the word means to them. Circulate memos and drafts. Sponsor informal lunchtime meetings among groups of employees to bat ideas around.

Only then should you consider taking a group of people offsite. The group should definitely include the chief executive and other C-level officers; it might also include a small but representative sample of professionals and other staff and of the board. When that group comes up with a draft, take it back to the other employees and the full board for a critique. It will not be long before you see a consensus emerging—and now it is a consensus that carries buy-in along with it, simply because so many people have their thumbprints on the process.

Constructing the Statement

There are some basic guidelines for the wording of a mission statement as well. Fundamentally, a mission statement is a promise. A good word when you are making a promise is we, as in "We commit ourselves..." or "We seek to...." The word we personalizes the statement and gives it a human touch; it suggests that real people are running the organization and that these people are personally committing themselves to accomplish something. It also makes the people who are writing the statement take it more seriously; few of us like to make a promise that we think we cannot keep. The promise—the statement—should be signed and dated by the CEO and board of directors or trustees. That commits the organization to staying the course.

The promise must be both meaningful and memorable. It should touch the heart and it should stick in the mind. It should get to the core of what the organization wants to be. It is not enough to say that you commit yourselves to the highest quality, for instance—what does that mean to the people you want your organization to serve? If trust is to be at the core of your mission, say that you commit yourselves to building trust, or to becoming the most trusted organization in your marketplace.

Finally, the statement must be brief. If brevity is the soul of wit, it is also the key to a statement that is meaningful and memorable. Ideally, it should be no longer than 25 words, and certainly no longer than 50. Albert Einstein once said, "Make everything as simple as possible, but not simpler." That rule applies to the mission statement. No one wants to read a laundry list of processes that they do not care about.

To get started, you may draw from the following list of frequently appearing words and phrases in mission statements:

- Organization is dedicated to (or exclusively dedicated to) providing/to provide: the finest; the highest quality; unsurpassed (to serving target population)...this commitment drives us to: (bulleted list)
- Organization's purpose is to (improve)
- Organization is dedicated to enhancing: lives; quality; profitability
- The mission of this organization is to serve; to be preeminent (in providing)

Figure 8.1. Mission Promise Worksheet

(Not all elements will be used by every organization.)

At____
[Name of organization]

we____
[Word of commitment, e.g., promise, aim]

to____
[Goal or goals of the organization]

by____
[Actions that will define organization in the marketplace and accomplish goals]

- Our mission is to provide (comprehensive) services/products through excellence and the continuous improvement of
- Through leadership and innovation organization will create solutions to (problems)
- Being a leading source
- To provide leadership (in the delivery of)
- Champions of
- To nurture, advance, and protect
- In order to restore, sustain, enhance...the (health)
- Advocates (for the rights of); an advocate on behalf of (target population)
- To educate, engage, lead, improve, restore (through the provision of...)
- To improve/dedicated to improving (something—e.g., health of children) through the provision of
- Dedicated to making
- Organization is committed to...by providing the finest possible
- Within our commitment to...we espouse
- Seeks to be/strives to be (mission or vision)

These phrases can be inserted into the mission promise worksheet shown in Figure 8.1.

This articulation of your reason for being will, if carefully composed and used, play a significant role in the future of your organization.

Living up to the Statement

How can a mission statement become a living, breathing force—a guide to action—rather than simply a collection of words on the wall? Ideally, the mission informs everything your organization does: how and whom it hires; how it interacts with employees, prospects, and customers; how it operates internally; how it launches new products and services; and more (see the box titled "Sample Mission Statements" for examples). If the mission statement defines a promise, after all, then all of these actions are simply ways of carrying out the promise.

This process can be formalized by an approach known as mission-based management (MBM). It tracks and manages resources on a mission-specific basis. Some member institutions of the Association of American Medical Colleges (AAMC) began using this approach in the 1999–2000 academic year (AAMC 2004). Leaders can make sure that the mission of the institution is fulfilled in its activities using data reporting and analysis. The first step is detailing the full mission of the institution. After dividing this mission into categories, measure the activity of various units or individuals in each category, as well as in financial performance, and then comparatively analyze the data.

The following are key features of MBM (adapted from AAMC 2004 and with permission by AAMC and David S. Hefner, Senior Partner, Computer Sciences Corporation):

1. *Integrating institutional financial statements.* Understanding the various costs and revenues associated with each mission helps organizations make strategic decisions and allocate resources effectively.
2. *Measuring individual and departmental activities and contributions to mission.* Compiling and tracking information about clinical and departmental activities and contributions clarifies organizational standards for accountability and expectations on overall performance.
3. *Building organizational support for reporting tools and metrics.* Using institutional design teams as the vehicle, leadership must

Sample Mission Statements

Children's Hospitals and Clinics champions the special health needs of children and their families.

We are committed to improving children's health by providing high-quality, family-centered pediatric services.

We advance these efforts through research and education.

—*Children's Hospitals and Clinics (Minneapolis/St. Paul)*

We are the eyes and ears of the nation and at times its hidden hand. We accomplish this mission by:

- Collecting intelligence that matters.
- Providing relevant, timely, and objective all-source analysis.
- Conducting covert action at the direction of the President to preempt threats or achieve United States policy objectives.

—*Central Intelligence Agency*

The Bettendorf Public Library Information Center is committed to providing access to information and ideas for all.

—*Bettendorf Public Library (Bettendorf, Iowa)*

We dedicate ourselves to humanity's quest for longer, healthier, happier lives through innovation in pharmaceutical, consumer, and animal health products.

—*Pfizer*

build a consensus on the specific metrics that will be used to measure clinical and departmental contributions within each mission.

4. *Guiding the dynamics of leadership.* Supported by dependable data, leaders are encouraged to engage in communication, and honest and open dialog with their colleagues. This dialog is particularly critical for the inevitably sensitive discussions about productivity and its relationship to the financial health of and scope of opportunities open to the institution.
5. *Holding key staff and department and institution leaders accountable.* Organizations need an effective procedure for

establishing their priorities and for holding departmental leaders accountable for meeting or exceeding expectations. The specifics as to how decisions are made and how accountability is ensured can take many forms, consistent with the leadership style and philosophy of the CEO.

6. *Building trust and institutional perspective.* Mission-based management affords the opportunity to share data and other information across departments and with key staff members. Open exploration of the facts establishes trust and encourages a broader vision of the enterprise as a whole. It also furnishes the organization's leaders with a rational, informed basis for aligning resources quickly and more accurately in response to the actual results produced by key staff members.

The "Mission-based Management Resource Materials Introductory Guide," produced by AAMC, provides a comprehensive overview of the AAMC Mission-based Management Program, an institutional readiness assessment survey, and an explanation of the MBM Resource Materials. MBM provides a starting point in examining your organization's mission and whether your resources and performance align with it.

At a minimum, it is worth continuing the discussions that led up to the mission statement, perhaps on a quarterly or semiannual basis. Are we doing what we said we would? Are we keeping our promise? These are powerful questions, and employees who are committed to the organization will take them very seriously. The discussions can provide senior management with a kind of reality check as to whether the mission is real in the only place where it can be real—the hearts and minds of those charged with carrying it out.

VISION

"Would you tell me, please, which way I ought to go from here?"
"That depends a good deal on where you want to get to," said the Cat.

"I don't much care where—" said Alice.
"Then it doesn't matter which way you go," said the Cat.
—Lewis Carroll, *Alice's Adventures in Wonderland*

Vision is a much used (and much overused) term, but it is indispensable to an organization seeking its direction. If mission spells out the organization's purpose, vision describes where it is going. What do you want the organization to become? Where do you want it to be in 10 or 20 years? Understanding vision is the second step in constructing a company's *raison d'être*. As you read the following sections describing what a vision entails, consider the statements in the box titled "Sample Vision Statements."

A Vision Looks Toward the Future

Nobody has a crystal ball, and nobody can forecast accurately. What organizations can do is set out a clear direction, an end point that serves as a touchstone. They can say *what they want to become* and *where they want to be*. A good vision bridges the present and the future by showing a path for going forward.

A Vision Inspires

Think about the grand visions of recent history. "Before the end of this decade, America will put a man on the moon," declared John F. Kennedy. "I have a dream," announced Rev. Martin Luther King, Jr., and proceeded to enumerate the many facets of his vision of equality and justice. A vision is a statement of aspirations, a target that beckons. It is by definition ambitious and grand, uplifting and ennobling. It creates meaning in stakeholders' lives because they have something to aspire to. It attracts people. It engenders energy, direction, and commitment. Further, the vision should not only spark the imagination, it should also be written in a fashion that

Sample Vision Statements

Our Vision: Become one of the nation's best pediatric providers, accessible to all children.

—Children's Hospitals and Clinics (Minneapolis/St. Paul)

We will provide knowledge and take action to ensure the national security of the United States and the preservation of American life and ideals.

—Central Intelligence Agency

The Bettendorf Public Library Information Center will be the recognized source of knowledge and information, the place to gather and discuss, the encourager of reading, and the leader in cooperation with the city, schools, and organizations.

We will be the gateway to lifelong learning, offering a full spectrum of services, materials, and programming.

—Bettendorf Public Library (Bettendorf, Iowa)

Our mission: We will become the world's most valued company to patients, customers, colleagues, investors, business partners, and the communities where we work and live.

—Pfizer

Note: the Pfizer statement is stated as mission, but it is actually a vision.

inspires. The language should be filled with passion and commitment. It should be evocative and compelling. The vision should reflect high ideals, but not be perceived as unattainable.

A Vision Instills Dynamism

No organization is on the verge of realizing its vision; if it is, the vision is too limited. An ambitious vision—one that projects a future that may be some years distant—allows the organization to benchmark its progress and to move toward the vision. It allows positioning promises to evolve over time as capacity increases and new challenges present themselves. Where you want to go may not be as important as where you end up, but having a perspective on where you want to go is the first step to getting closer to it. A vision is a yardstick by which to gauge progress.

A Vision Is a Key Element of Leadership

Vision is a central element in Theodore Roosevelt's advice to leaders, as summarized in the four guidelines below (Strock 2001):

1. Craft and present a compelling vision.
2. Reframe the discussion in terms that advance your vision.
3. Set and enforce priorities for the achievement of the vision.
4. Implement the "theory of the next step."

In short, it is a leader's job to establish the vision and relate the steps an organization can take now—the next steps—to the ultimate destination. There is little that is more important. As with mission, however, a vision developed collectively is even more powerful than one handed down by a leader. Employees can enrich the vision of an organization well past the boundaries set by its founders. And they are more likely to buy into and be inspired by a vision that bears their own fingerprints. The vision will be shared, right from the start. Use the vision promise worksheet shown in Figure 8.2 to begin developing the vision statement for your organization.

VALUES

I have saved values for last, because many organizations already know what they value and need only to build a mission and a vision on that foundation. But is your organization one of those that knows its values? Have they been made explicit? Do they appear in company communications, from the annual report to the web site? If not, you will have to begin here and establish your values before

Figure 8.2. Vision Promise Worksheet

To become the____
[Adjective similar to best or leading]

in____
[Market category]

known for____
[Organization's aspirations]

by all of our____
[Target market(s)]

considering mission and vision. A useful technique is to sponsor small-group workshops in which you ask people to write down the values that they personally hold dear and specify which of those values they believe should lie at the heart of the organization. Follow much the same iterative procedure as for mission and vision, involving people throughout the organization (especially including board members and senior executives) until a consensus emerges.

As with mission and vision statements, the written values statement should be brief: 5 values are far better than 25. Limiting your statement to five values helps you effectively and efficiently communicate them. And understand that—unlike mission and vision, which must reflect an organization's changing circumstances over time—values should virtually never change. As former IBM CEO Thomas Watson, Jr., put it, "The only sacred cow in an organization should be its basic philosophy of doing business" (Watson 2003).

Finally, there is no fixed recipe for coming up with a statement of values, nor for writing them down. However, there are guidelines to begin constructing your values statement. Many organizations use a list to convey their values. It is more effective to personalize it, as with the phrase "Our values." Following the idea of the values statement, consider displaying the longevity of your commitment: "We will always value diversity." Begin with an overarching value if you have one, and then add others that are supportive of it: "We will always do what is best for each child." If possible, you may wish to link the values statement to your mission and vision: "We put our customers first by (insert values)."

Generally, the core values emphasized in organizational values statements (see the box titled "Sample Values Statements" for examples) fall into three main categories. In one category, the organization

Sample Values Statements

The ProHealth Promise™

We believe that our first responsibility is to our patients. Everything we do must be with their health and well-being in mind. We will build lasting relationships with patients and their families based on trust, mutual respect, and integrity. We will advocate for our patients and serve as their primary resource to maintain their health. We will work in partnership with our patients to achieve the best medical care that is right for them.

We believe in the importance of health promotion and disease prevention. We dedicate ourselves to outstanding care and excellent service. We support research and education that improves the health of our patients. We are open to new ideas, and we are committed to improving our skills and knowledge.

We are all members of the same ProHealth Team working together with a common purpose. We will treat each other with respect, understanding, and appreciation for the merit of each individual. We believe in the value of team work and collaboration. We are committed to developing the skills and potential of each person in ProHealth Physicians. We will foster a work place that is positive, creative, and dedicated to the health of the people we serve.

We will work together to sustain, improve, and grow a healthy organization that has the needed resources to accomplish all of our goals.

We will bring honesty, integrity, trust and value to our relationships with other healthcare professionals and business partners.

We support the communities in which we work and live. We will help to improve the public health and well being.

When we keep this Promise in our work each day, we can fulfill our mission to improve the lives of all those we serve.

—Adopted by ProHealth Physicians – Spring 2004

(continued on the following page)

Sample Values Statements *(continued)*

Our Promise:
The Department of Surgery at New York Hospital Queens provides our patients with optimal care while at the same time is attentive to their physical, psychological, and cultural needs.

We are committed to our patients by providing excellent care while maintaining their dignity and treating them with respect and compassion. We continuously educate our patients and their families so they can work collaboratively with their health care providers in making decisions that affect their health.

We are committed to our colleagues by encouraging them to develop both personally and professionally. We are dedicated to educating our students, faculty, and staff, in order to continually increase the knowledge and skills required for excellent care. Our organization promotes an environment of trust and recognizes the importance of collaboration in providing the best patient care.

We are committed to promoting continuous quality improvement and expanding our services in order to satisfy the changing needs of our culturally diverse community.

—*New York Hospital Queens Department of Surgery*

indicates that it meets the needs and exceeds the expectations of every person/customer. In another, it describes its recruitment and support of highly skilled, caring people. In a third category, the organization describes its efforts to establish meaningful relationships with all stakeholders.

In my research, I have found additional specific values that are frequently cited in values statements. The most common ones are listed below in order of frequency of appearance.

1. Quality
2. Innovation
3. Teamwork
4. Honesty
5. Integrity
8. Financial responsiblity
9. Efficient and effective resource use
10. Customer service
11. Diversity
12. Advocacy

6. Excellence
7. Leadership
13. Advocacy
14. Charity

Your organization can develop its statement from the above guidelines or develop something all its own, as did Johnson & Johnson. Probably the most powerful values statement in American business today is the famous Credo of Johnson & Johnson, and in many respects it breaks all the rules. It was articulated by Gen. Robert Wood Johnson, not developed through a participatory process. It is

Our Credo

We believe our first responsibility is to the doctors, nurses and patients, to mothers and fathers and all others who use our products and services. In meeting their needs everything we do must be of high quality. We must constantly strive to reduce our costs in order to maintain reasonable prices. Customers' orders must be serviced promptly and accurately. Our suppliers and distributors must have an opportunity to make a fair profit.

We are responsible to our employees, the men and women who work with us throughout the world. Everyone must be considered as an individual. We must respect their dignity and recognize their merit. They must have a sense of security in their jobs. Compensation must be fair and adequate, and working conditions clean, orderly and safe.
We must be mindful of ways to help our employees fulfill their family responsibilities. Employees must feel free to make suggestions and complaints. There must be equal opportunity for employment, development and advancement for those qualified. We must provide competent management, and their actions must be just and ethical.

We are responsible to the communities in which we live and work and to the world community as well. We must be good citizens support good works and charities and bear our fair share of taxes. We must encourage civic improvements and better health and education. We must maintain in good order the property we are privileged to use, protecting the environment and natural resources.

Our final responsibility is to our stockholders. Business must make a sound profit. We must experiment with new ideas. Research must be carried on, innovative programs developed and mistakes paid for. New equipment must be purchased, new facilities provided and new products launched. Reserves must be created to provide for adverse times. When we operate according to these principles, the stockholders should realize a fair return.

lengthy, it incorporates elements of mission and vision as well as values, and it has been updated modestly over the years to reflect changing times. Still, it has served as a reference point, guide, and touchstone for this superb company for more than 60 years—never so much as when the company faced the Tylenol crises of 1982 and 1986 (see Chapter 9, "The Deed or the Cover-up"). "With Johnson & Johnson's good name and reputation at stake," the company says on its web site, "company managers and employees made countless decisions that were inspired by the philosophy embodied in the Credo" (Johnson & Johnson).

So read the Johnson & Johnson Credo in the box on page 118 not as a blueprint but as one possible approach an organization can take to establishing its values, noting how thorough and explicit a statement of values it is.

A credo such as this governs the hearts and minds of Johnson & Johnson. It aligns people with goals, provides meaning, and motivates people to stretch and grow. It provides an organizational *raison d'être*, which in turn is the basis for establishing a company's reputation.

REFERENCES

Association of American Medical Colleges. 2004. "Mission-based Management Archive." [Online information; retrieved 11/22/04.] http://www .aamc.org /members/msmr/mbmapproach.htm.

Johnson & Johnson. http://www.jnj.com/our_company/our_credo_history.

MeaningfulWorkplace.com. 2000. "Employee Insight Survey." [Online survey results; retrieved 11/22/04.] http://www.meaningfulworkplace.com/survey.

Oleck, J. 1998. "Footnotes." *Business Week* 3601: 8.

Strock, J. M. 2001. *Theodore Roosevelt on Leadership: Executive Lessons from the Bully Pulpit* 162–76. Roseville, CA: Prima Publishing.

Watson, T. J. 2003. *A Business and Its Beliefs: The Ideas that Helped Build IBM*, 73. New York: McGraw-Hill.

CHAPTER NINE

The Building Blocks: Increasing Your Trust Capacity

Trust is built in many steps and can be destroyed in one.

—*Eric Hoffer*

WHAT, YOU MAY be asking, does all of this talk about power brands and *raison d'être* have to do with trust? The question will be answered in this chapter. To begin, let us revisit Doug, the plumber.

A few years have passed. By now you and Doug have come to know each other well. He fixed the first leaky pipe competently and billed you for an amount you thought was fair. Later you called him to fix a different leak—aren't old houses wonderful?—and then to install a new heating system. His estimate on the heating system was right on the money, and, in general, you were highly pleased with the installation.

One cold night, however, the bedroom was freezing, and you discovered there was no heat in the entire second floor. You called him at six o'clock in the morning. He was there by seven. In half an hour he had found the problem: a defective pump. "I made a mistake," he told you. "I installed a pump I bought from a new supplier, and I didn't know whether it was reliable. I'm sorry. I'll replace it with a new pump free of charge."

Impressed, you have since asked him back to redo a bathroom, a $10,000 job. The work was superb. You begin recommending him to friends. You have started to ask after his family, and he after yours. You have given him a key to the house so that you can ask him to do things while you are away.

What you are feeling toward Doug is no longer just "trust" in the ordinary sense. It might better be called *deep personal trust.* We have all felt this kind of trust in close friends and members of our families. Most of us have felt it in the occasional tradesperson, professional, store owner, or institution. Some of us feel deep personal trust in our physician or health center. We say things like, "I would trust her with my life," or "I know I can always rely on them to do the right thing."

Deep personal trust is both rational and emotive—both left brain and right brain. Residing in the left brain, the seat of reason, are our cognitive assessments of other people. We deduce that we can trust them based on their actions in the past. In the right brain are all of the emotional components of trust: an affective belief that other people have our best interests at heart, a liking for them, and a feeling of comfort and confidence. Deep personal trust comprises logic and love, not logic or love.

Deep personal trust most often begins with a personal relationship. But note that it is not always just one human being to another. Suppose Doug the plumber sent an experienced journeyman to do some of the work; chances are you would have confidence in that plumber as well. Similarly, you may know and trust your accountant or lawyer as an individual, but your trust probably includes the bank or law firm that they work for as well. This halo effect is critically important for the people who run organizations. The reason is that organizations, too, can develop their *trust capacity*—the capacity to engender deep personal trust in the people whose lives the organization touches. A trusted organization is trusted by its customers or patients, its employees and professional staff, its suppliers, its investors or donors, and its community.

Here, then, is where trust comes together with what we have been discussing. An organization that sees itself in the trust business—an organization that wants to build a power brand around trust—needs a mission and a vision that lay out that objective. The organization's leaders and employees must commit themselves to occupying the trust space in the marketplace. But that involves much more than simply crafting the right wording on a statement and launching a marketing campaign around trust. It involves building the organization's trust capacity so that it can in fact act in a way that develops trust. It involves operationalizing the mission and vision so that trust is built into the bone and sinew of the organization's day-to-day activity.

Trust, however, is not a single entity. Developing your trust capacity is more like assembling a structure out of building blocks, each one depending on the others to create an edifice. Trust is constructed one block at a time.

THE TRUST DEVELOPMENT MODEL: COMPETENCE

There are probably a dozen cues that inspire trust, and not all of them are subject to management. If you are the producer of Guinness, the well-known Irish stout, you can keep on reminding your customers that you have been making it since 1759. Longevity is a great trust builder. If you are Wal-Mart stores, you can tell your customers that you have grown to be the largest retailer in the world in just a few decades. Most healthcare providers and organizations—a nursing service at a community hospital, a regional managed care company—cannot make such grand claims because they do not happen to be the oldest, the biggest, or most in whatever category. What they can do is focus their efforts on the many other trustworthiness cues that matter to consumers.

The cornerstones are the fundamental components of trust described in Chapter 1, competence and conscience. Consumers come to healthcare with high expectations. They expect physicians and other professionals to know their jobs, treat their patients warmly and sympathetically, and never make an error. They expect healthcare organizations to operate efficiently, effectively, and humanely. They also expect everyone in the healthcare enterprise to have their—the patients'—best interests at heart.

Competence is about credibility: it determines to what extent patients believe that providers or organizations have the skills and experience to perform effectively and reliably. It is about the *care that you give.* Conscience, by contrast, is about benevolence, the extent to which patients believe that providers and organizations have motives beneficial to patients. Conscience is about the *caring that you show.* Trusted clinicians—indeed, trusted healthcare professionals and organizations of all sorts—contribute to patients' well-being through competent advice, responsible treatment, and compassionate care.

Let us consider the competence component of trust first, by examining some of its key elements: capacity, credibility, confidence, and consistency.

Capacity

No provider or organization can do everything. But what can you do? What do you do? The capacity building block entails knowing exactly what your mission is and offering programs, products, or services that further that mission. It entails giving the consumer clear descriptions of what you can and will do, as well as explaining (when necessary) what you cannot or will not do.

This seems like a simple lesson. But how many physicians think that they have all of the answers and can treat every patient? How many hospitals try to have all the latest equipment even though they may not have the scope or the expertise necessary to utilize it efficiently? How many nursing homes take in patients that they cannot effectively care for? To understand and communicate your capacity is to understand where you can add value and further your mission and where you cannot. It is to respect the limitations of any single organization and the human beings who make it up.

Credibility

Trust depends not only on what you promise—what you can do—but also on whether you deliver on your promises. All the capacity in the world means little if your customers and other stakeholders do not believe that you can deliver. Credibility thus depends on your performance. Remember, too, that performance in a healthcare setting includes virtually every aspect that a customer or stakeholder might be able to judge. It includes clean bathrooms as well as successful surgeries. It includes friendly accounts receivable staff as well as top-quality physician services (see the box titled "Eliminate the Trustbusters"). Customers of managed care companies are likely to judge the organization both by how long it takes them to answer the telephone and then by how long it takes to get an answer to a question.

Confidence

The companion of credibility, of course, is confidence: the comforting feeling that you are in good hands. Confidence in healthcare is not simply a matter of warm and fuzzy feelings; it affects outcomes. Cardiologist Herbert Benson, M.D., president of the Mind/Body Medical Institute in Chestnut Hill, Massachusetts, has shown that if a patient has confidence in his or her physician and/or the recommended treatment and if in turn the physician expresses confidence in the treatment plan, the patient's chance of healing can be improved by 60 to 80 percent (Benson 1997). Patient-physician belief and confidence in the treatment are part of a larger phenomenon Dr. Benson calls "remembered wellness," and it is a powerful one. Equally powerful is the loss of such confidence and belief, which usually causes the gains to be reversed (Benson 1997).

Eliminate the Trustbusters

Building trust capacity is hard work, and all of your effort can be undermined by simple trustbusters, or proxies. Proxies are nonclinical criteria that consumers and patients use in evaluating healthcare providers and organizations, because it is difficult for them to evaluate the highly complex and technical practice of medicine and medical administration.

The top five proxies are as follows:

1. Dirty bathrooms or overflowing trash cans. "If they cannot even keep the bathroom (or hallways) clean, how do I know that the operating room will be clean?"
2. Errors in billing. "If they cannot even get the bill right, how do I know if I got the right prescription?"
3. Rudeness or abruptness on the part of receptionists, administrators, physicians, and anybody else. People enter the healthcare system feeling anxious and vulnerable. They need reassurance, not rudeness.
4. Inconsistencies of all sorts. In admissions: "That's not what I had to do last time." In clinical contexts: "Dr. Jones never said I had to do that." In insurance: "Last time the copay was only $10," or "Last time I was covered for this procedure."
5. Misplaced priorities. The receptionist who asks for the insurance card before saying, "How can we help you?"; the physician who ignores today's complaint while asking detailed questions about last month's; the nursing home that shows visitors its lovely garden while ignoring the smell of urine in the hallways.

Consistency

The bane of every service organization is the situation when a customer gets great service one day, or at one location, and gets terrible service the next day, or at another location. Service companies from McDonald's to the Ritz-Carlton hotel chain establish precise standards for service and train their employees accordingly. Healthcare, of course, is more challenging than most other service industries put together. The stakes are higher, and the problems are more complex.

Every job is a custom job because every patient is different, every presenting problem is different, every clinician is different, every claim is different. Still, healthcare organizations cannot afford variability in their standards of service, if only because consumers tend to focus more on one negative experience than on a dozen positive ones. The many initiatives relating to quality of service that hospitals are now undertaking serve more than anything else to boost consistency.

Consistency has two other dimensions as well. One is consistency of message over time, where "time" may be a period of years or decades. Volvo has repeated its safety message for so long that "Volvo" and "safety" are inextricably linked in the minds of car buyers. Disney's anniversary slogan, "100 Years of Magic," reminds consumers that the company has been engaged in magical entertainment for longer than most people have lived. Trusted brands—and trusted healthcare providers or organizations—are always what they say they are, and they do not change that message from one year to the next. This fact highlights the need for careful planning at the beginning of the brand-building process. Once you embark on building a brand around trust, you have made a long-term commitment.

Another dimension of consistency is continuity. About a decade ago, the Institute of Medicine (IOM) defined *primary care* as "the provision of integrated, accessible health care services by clinicians who are accountable for addressing a large majority of personal health needs, *developing a sustained partnership with patients* [italics added], and practicing in the context of family and community." The salient phrase here, which did not appear in the earlier (1978) definition, is "sustained partnership." IOM determined that continuity of the primary care relationship is central.[1] By extension, it is also central to building trust. Continuity represents a commitment to the patient that the organization is going to be there tomorrow and the next day and the day after that. It is more difficult to trust an unknown and transitory organization or individual, because there is no basis to do so. Continuity is a commitment to stick with a location, an organization, a group of patients, or other continuation of business. It also entails knowing the target community and the patients well, and showing it, whether by remembering Mrs. Smith's name and case or by participating in community outreach efforts.

Commitment

A healthcare provider or organization has choices. It can take a passive approach to its business, in effect operating on the assumption that it is doing its best, or it can take a more active approach, focusing on ways to improve its performance. It can also take a passive approach to its patients, waiting for them to walk in the door, or it can practice "outbound" healthcare, seeking people out and offering them information and services that they may need. Imagine that a patient undergoes surgery at hospital A. All she receives from the hospital after the surgery is a bill or a copy of the charges that the hospital has sent to the insurance company. Then imagine a similar patient at hospital B. Instead of just a bill, she receives a follow-up visit (perhaps at her home), some informational material on recovering from this particular kind of surgery, and health-related news tailored to people in her situation. How different will the two patients' feelings be toward their hospital?

The degree to which a hospital or other healthcare organization is proactive in this way reflects its commitment to building trust. Typically, after all, the entire healthcare enterprise is "out of sight, out of mind" to patients unless they are sick or injured. The proactive, committed organization is not out of sight, hence not out of mind. It is always there. It is more likely to be trusted and chosen again and again.

THE TRUST DEVELOPMENT MODEL: CONSCIENCE

Competence alone is not a differentiator in the marketplace. It is more of an entry ticket to the marketplace. In healthcare, consumers take it for granted, not surprisingly, as it is heavily regulated by federal and state governments and medical professional societies. But if competence is the basic expectation on the part of patients, conscience is the value-added attribute that they seek out. Like competence, the conscience side of trust can be divided into a handful of building blocks. Many of them are easily described, if not always easy to live up to.

Character, for example, refers simply to integrity. It can be said (perhaps cynically) that character is how you behave when you know you can get away with something. This is a central issue in healthcare, because patients are so often unable to see or judge what healthcare professionals do. Physicians who find clever ways to defraud Medicare or who perform procedures that are not necessary flunk the character test. Hospitals that try to cover up their errors flunk it, too. Doctors who cave in to HMO pressures to limit necessary care also fail. "Watch your thoughts; they become words," quoted by Frank Outlaw; "watch your words; they become actions. Watch your actions; they become habits. Watch your habits; they become character. Watch your character; it becomes your destiny."[2] It is as true of organizations as it is of individuals.

Compassion, similarly, refers to the caring shown by the provider toward the patient. In a hospital, think of the difference between a physician who stands stiffly in the doorway of the patient's room, one foot already in the corridor, and the one who sits in a chair near the bed. In a managed care organization, imagine what it would mean if a physician or nurse came out into the waiting room to greet the member, sat on the couch chatting for a moment or two, and then escorted the member into the examining room. The simple human qualities of warmth, empathy, and genuineness underscore a provider's compassion toward a fellow human being who is sick, in pain, or simply anxious and uncertain. Because healthcare deals with such situations every day, it cannot operate effectively without compassion.

Other of these building blocks, including community, consumer focus, and communication, are discussed at more length in the following sections.

Community

When IOM added the phrase "sustained partnership with patients" to its definition of primary care, it also added another: "practicing in the context of family and community" (IOM 1994). This is a high-sounding phrase that might be just a meaningless platitude. But in medicine it has a very specific meaning: familiarity. Consumers and patients want their clinicians to be intimately familiar with their situation. They crave some degree of connectedness, closeness, or intimacy with the treatment team. They want to be part of this small community, rather than feeling like a faceless individual treated just like everybody else.

Familiarity derives from the same root as family, and it is precisely that family feeling that patients want. The Olive Garden restaurant chain promises its customers, "When you're here, you're family." Can a healthcare organization promise any less? Every doctor, nurse, and pharmacist has heard the question, "What would you do if it were your child?" or "What would you do if it were your mother?" Patients want to feel that they get the same treatment as a provider's family member and that they experience the same level of comfort and trust as if the provider were a family member.

Consumer Focus

Many factors have contributed to today's world of consumer-driven healthcare. The recent trend for insurance plans to be less restrictive than they were in the 1990s has given consumers more choice. Consumers have access to more information, as we have seen. They are being asked to play a growing role in medical decisions and processes. It all makes some sense, because patients—particularly those with chronic illnesses—are critical members of their own care team. But many healthcare organizations have not yet understood all of the implications of a true consumer focus. Consumers want *convenience*. They want access at different times of day or night, with options for full-time, around-the-clock access through the Internet or the telephone. They want *convergence*—a seamless system, under one roof, that integrates clinical care, medication, and payment—the medical version of one-stop shopping. They want *collaboration*—not only between them and their physician but also among all the healthcare providers that care for them. The disparate collection of providers and payers that make up the healthcare enterprise has generally collaborated poorly. Genuine collaborative efforts would go far toward engendering trust. One example of such an effort is when managed care organizations hire dedicated provider representatives for each provider to improve collaboration between the two. In addition, managed care companies often hire affiliated physicians to serve on credentialing and medical services review committees, further developing the relationship. When collaboration improves, all stakeholders benefit.

Communication

Trust and communication go hand in glove: open communication encourages trust, and trust facilitates communication. Trusted clinician-patient communication enhances diagnosis, treatment, and compliance. Still, communication in healthcare typically runs into a series of obstacles related to listening, clarity, and confidentiality.

Listening is as important to communication as talking. Yet many physicians are not good listeners, if only because they do not take the time to hear what patients are trying to put into words. Healthcare organizations, insurance companies, and pharmaceutical manufacturers are notoriously poor listeners. Virtually every customer of these institutions could delineate a litany of complaints related to poor listening. Few organizations have established a channel for listening to complaints and taking them seriously.

Clarity is also an issue. Doctors may speak in medical jargon. They may force-feed a patient too much information or starve the patient with too little. Some physicians fall back on the notion that they just are not good communicators; the patient would be better off just doing what they say, and never mind all the explanation. Ninety million people, or 47 percent of the U.S. population, are categorized by IOM as having limited health literacy (Neilson-Bohlman, Panzer, and Kindig 2004). The U.S. Department of Health and Human Services defines health literacy as "The degree to which individuals have the capacity to obtain, process, and understand basic health information and services needed to make appropriate health decisions" (Ratzan and Parker 2000). The challenge for physicians is deciding what information to impart and how to impart it. The physician should at least ask if the patient understands the information, and the patient has a responsibility to communicate uncertainty or trepidation. Clarity is a team effort.

Confidentiality can be another obstacle to good communication. Patients are fiercely protective of their privacy. Yet collaborative healthcare requires sharing of information among clinicians and other interested parties. Confidentiality and collaboration are always in tension and must be balanced.

REGAINING LOST TRUST

How many institutions and organizations have recently watched whatever trust they had built up over the years simply vanish? How many others have seen their reputation for probity and quality plummet? The shortest of lists would certainly include the following:

- Major corporations, including Enron, Tyco, Global Crossing, and WorldCom, which saw their stock value evaporate and their very survival threatened because of malfeasance in the top ranks
- The Catholic Church, rocked by serious allegations of repeated sexual abuse of children by priests, in many cases without apparent punitive consequences for the erring priests or the Church itself

- The once-venerable accounting firm Arthur Andersen, which was liquidated when it appeared that the firm would never be able to regain clients' trust in the wake of the Enron scandal
- *The New York Times*, which discovered that a young journalist who had been nurtured and promoted by senior editors was in fact fabricating many facts in his stories, leading eventually to the forced resignation of the paper's top two editors

These and many other scandals, of course, came in the wake of highly publicized trustbusters attributed to U.S. presidents, and in healthcare, the collapse of Richard Scrushy's HealthSouth empire was only the most visible of a series of well-reported trustbusting scandals.

Scandals and other trust crises tend to follow a similar pattern. Typically, allegations of wrongdoing appear in the news media. Leaders of the institution in question deny the allegations and meanwhile launch an internal effort to cover up whatever wrongdoing occurred. If possible, they blame somebody else, as when Firestone and Ford fueded over who was responsible in response to charges that Firestone tires were leading to fatal accidents involving Ford's Explorer vehicles. They continue denying the allegations right up to the point where it is no longer possible to do so—and finally they take steps to make the crisis go away, preferably without admitting culpability. *The New York Times* admitted in a front-page story the transgressions of its young reporter, but no one at the top of the paper took responsibility for the malfeasance until forced to do so by the continuing scandal. The Boston Archdiocese of the Catholic Church took months to get rid of the cardinal on whose watch much of the abuse there had taken place; the archbishop who succeeded the cardinal promptly settled the outstanding lawsuits for millions of dollars.

What is astonishing about all such trustbusting scandals is how regular the response pattern is, and how wrongheaded. There will always be threats to the trust that an organization has built up, simply because every organization is staffed by human beings and sometimes human beings will do the wrong thing. But these threats do not need to lead to an evaporation of trust; on the contrary, they can help build trust.

THE DEED OR THE COVER-UP?

Healthcare organizations face trust-threatening situations all the time. A doctor makes a mistake, and a patient's health or life is threatened. A hospital fails to treat a seriously ill patient correctly, and the patient dies. A pharmaceutical company experiences quality problems in its manufacturing. An HMO incorrectly denies a patient treatment for which he or she is covered. If it is bad enough, any such event is likely to wind up on the front page of the local newspaper. The real question is, what happens next?

"Americans tend to be a forgiving lot," wrote Ronald Alsop (2003) in *The Wall Street Journal*, "when companies confess their sins and do their penance." But little makes people angrier than when an organization seems to be stonewalling, denying the obvious and refusing to admit responsibility. Owning up to errors, mistakes, and miscalculations actually engenders trust, while denying them erodes trust even further. In short, you do not get into trouble for the deed, you get into trouble for the cover-up. From the Watergate scandal that broke in 1973, when it was the Nixon administration's repeated denial that eventually led to the president's resignation, to Martha Stewart, who was convicted not for insider trading but for lying about her involvement in it, the lesson has been the same: an organization's reputation is often more affected by the response than by the crisis itself.

This fact leads to some obvious, but sadly ignored, advice about how to deal with a trust-threatening occurrence.

1. Act quickly. Most of the damage to an organization's reputation occurs during the early phases of a crisis.
2. Say something. Silence is self-defeating. In an era of mistrust, silence is interpreted by the public as evidence of lack of concern

and an evasive attitude. It merely confirms the organization's lack of integrity in the public's eyes.

3. Say you are sorry. Apologize.
4. Take public steps to address the situation that caused the problem so that it does not happen again.

The best-known crisis in modern healthcare may be the Tylenol scares in 1982 and 1986, when capsules of the popular pain reliever were laced with cyanide, causing the death of seven people. In what has become a textbook case of the right way to respond to a crisis, Johnson & Johnson instantly recalled Tylenol from the shelves; eventually it discontinued the capsule form of the medicine and introduced "tamper-evident" packaging so that consumers would know if the bottle they purchased had been opened. The company spared no expense—it ended up taking a $100 million charge against earnings—and kept no secrets, announcing all of its moves quickly and publicly. The result was a temporary dip in Johnson & Johnson's reputation and stock value, both of which quickly returned to their former heights (Tedlow and Smith 1989). Incredibly, institutions today have not learned these lessons; too many still believe that they can somehow cover up their problems.

THE CONSUMER'S RESPONSE

Trust capacity is based on two promises: a promise of competence, and a promise of conscience. Building trust capacity means honoring those promises. Trust is something that we create, build, maintain, and sustain. At their best, healthcare organizations can assume the role of trusted advisor to consumers. They can become the people to whom consumers or patients turn when they need help and advice.

How much would that be worth? As any homeowner will tell you, the feeling that you have a plumber that you can trust is worth a lot of money. As any patient will tell you, the feeling that you have a physician or healthcare organization that you can trust is priceless. Trusting consumers feel confidence and comfort. They ensure continuity of care because they are loyal to the trusted provider or organization. Recall from Chapter 3 that trust is the top predictor of loyalty to a physician's practice. Consumers who trust are also compliant, which is to say that they are more likely to take their medicines, follow their regimens, and share their information fully. Building up trust capacity thus makes for more effective healthcare and more satisfied patients. That combination is difficult to beat.

NOTE

1. Defining Primary Care: An Interim Report. An interim report by a committee of the Institute of Medicine, Division of Health Care Services. Molla Donaldson, Karl Yordy, and Neal Vanselow, editors. National Academy Press. October 1994. p. 1.
2. This quote succinctly sums up the importance of character in running a healthcare organization. Note that I was unable to confirm author attribution.

REFERENCES

Alsop, R. 2003. "Scandal-filled Year Takes Toll on Companies' Good Names." *Wall Street Journal* March 12, B1.

Benson, H. 1997. *Timeless Healing*. New York: Scribner.

Nielson-Bohlman, L., A. M. Panzer, and D. A. Kindig (eds.). 2004. *Health Literacy: A Prescription to End Confusion*. Washington, DC: The National Academies Press.

Ratzan, S. C., and R. M. Parker. 2000. "Introduction." In *National Library of Medicine Current Bibliographies in Medicine: Health Literacy*, edited by C. R. Seldon, M. Zorn, S. C. Ratzan, and R. M. Parker. NLM Pub. No. CBM 2000-1. Bethesda, MD: U.S. Department of Health and Human Services.

Tedlow, R. S., and W. K. Smith. 1989. "James Burke: A Career in American Business (B)." Harvard Business School Case #9-390-030. Boston: Harvard Business School.

CHAPTER TEN

A Reputation—and a Position—Based on Trust

> A company's value today may amount to its "capitalized reputation."
>
> —*Alan Greenspan*

THE FIRST PHASE in developing a brand around trust is to look inward: to take that voyage into the heart and soul of the organization and come up with a mission, vision, and set of values that truly capture who you are. If your mission, vision, and values revolve around trust, you must then put your organization's trust capacity to the test. A power brand based on trust is not simply a marketing statement; it is a statement about your entire organization, about who you are and what you do. Just as Volvo devotes millions of dollars and employee hours to improving its cars' safety performance, you must devote resources to improving your organization's trust performance. If you cannot be trusted, you cannot build a reputation based on trust.

But then comes the second phase: becoming *known* for trust, establishing a *position in the marketplace* around trust, and building a *reputation* that is based on trust. This second phase involves looking outward rather than inward, viewing things from the consumer's or patient's perspective rather than that of the organization. It entails creating a sustainable, defendable position in the marketplace, a position that is different from anybody else's. In this chapter we will examine the specifics of reputation—what it means (and does not mean) in the marketplace—and how you can create that reputation as the organization that can be trusted.

WHAT REPUTATION IS, AND WHY IT MATTERS

Reputation in everyday terminology typically refers to a thumbs-up or thumbs-down assessment of someone: a good reputation or a poor one. But reputation in the marketplace is a broader concept. Organizations occupy complex positions in consumers' minds. They engender a certain amount of positive or negative feeling. They stand for something that is somehow different from what other organizations in the same market category stand for. For the purposes of this discussion, then, *reputation* is the consensus of perceptions about how an organization will behave based on what people already know—or think they know—about that organization (Sandberg 2002).

Reputation has always been important in the business world in general, and of course in healthcare as well. We do business with a company that has a good reputation because we believe we can trust it to do what it says it will do. We visit doctors and hospitals with good reputations because we believe we can safely entrust our health to them. But note a critical difference here. When we go to the supermarket, we can assess the quality and prices of what we are buying with our own eyes. We may visit a store for the first time because it has a good reputation, but we visit it a second time primarily because we found that the quality and value were acceptable or superior. We ultimately make our judgments based on *tangible* factors. So it is with much of the economy. When it comes to clothes, appliances, automobiles, or computers, the reputation of the manufacturer matters. But it does not matter as much as the tangible value (or lack of value) that we eventually see in the goods themselves.

The service sector is different. When we hire a plumber, engage a lawyer, or entrust our life savings to a financial services firm, there is much that we do not and cannot know about the transaction. Does the person or company on the other end have our best interests at heart? Are they competent to do what we expect them to do? Do we know everything that we need to know about them? Most of us cannot easily assess the professional expertise of a plumber or lawyer, nor can we measure the stability of a financial services firm. In making a judgment about them, we are utterly dependent on their reputation.

More and more of our economy fits into this category, for good and for ill, because the marketplace has grown so much more complex over the years. Enron in its glory days was known for innovative contracts relating to the buying and selling of energy and other commodities; it had a reputation for being at the cutting edge of these markets and for doing things that no other company knew how to do. When the house-of-cards reality was finally exposed, Enron's old reputation collapsed—and suddenly it had a new reputation for double dealing and criminality. Its value, of course, collapsed along with its reputation. That is what Federal Reserve Bank chairman Alan Greenspan meant when he suggested that a company's value in many cases is no more than its capitalized reputation. Unlike General Motors, say, Enron had few tangible assets—factories, machinery, and so on—that would retain their value even if the company itself went under. When Enron's reputation dissolved, so did *all* of the company's value.

William Shakespeare wrote in *Richard II*, "The purest treasure mortal times afford/Is spotless reputation; that away,/Men are but gilded loam or painted clay." A modern-day Shakespeare might say as much about companies such as Enron.

There may be no industry in which reputation is as important as it is in healthcare. The stakes for a patient, after all, are huge, much larger than when that same person is purchasing a new suit of clothes. And the veil of ignorance hanging over their decisions is very nearly opaque. Patients can judge a doctor's manner, but they can rarely judge his or her professional competence and expertise. They can assess how clean a hospital's hallways are, but they can rarely assess whether its equipment is up to date and whether its procedures and protocols are state of the art. They can assess how a medication makes them feel (sometimes), but they cannot assess whether it was manufactured to the exact required specifications, nor can they easily assess the risk of undesirable side-effects. For all these judgments they are completely dependent on the reputation of the organization in question. Reputation becomes, in effect, a proxy for the quality that they are unable to judge.

That is why it can be reasonably said that the three most important words in developing a brand in healthcare are reputation, reputation, and reputation. "A good reputation is more valuable than money," observed the Roman slave and philosopher Publius Syrus in the first century B.C. The observation remains true practically as well as ethically: in healthcare, at least, a good reputation will generate business, but money alone cannot replace a good reputation.

ESTABLISHING A REPUTATION

A campaign to establish a reputation has two objectives. The first is to create a "mental location," a piece of real estate in the minds of the people who make up the target market. You want your reputation to be known by these people, to be part of their mental consideration set when they are making decisions about healthcare. The second is to create a reputation that carries with it what marketers like to call a unique selling proposition. Your objective is to differentiate yourself from the competition around something that your target market values. That makes your location unique in the mind of the market. Taken together, the two objectives will provide your organization with positioning in the sense described in Chapter 7. It will stand for something in the marketplace—something that is different from its competitors.

How to do it? At least three steps are involved: market research, research on the competition, and operational assessment.

Market Research

What does your marketplace want? Where is it underserved? Companies in many industries have choices about what position they set out to occupy. A donut chain may cultivate theatricality and panache, as Krispy Kreme has done with its stores, which allow customers to watch donuts being made and to buy them hot off the line. Or it may trade primarily on convenience, locating as many stores as possible in its target marketplace, as has been Dunkin' Donuts's chief strategy.

In healthcare, the situation is both similar and different. Healthcare organizations, too, always have choices. They may tout their convenience or their high-quality customer service. They may position themselves as experts in certain kinds of illness or injury. The range of options, however, is limited by the nature of the industry. For example, nobody is likely to want "bargain" healthcare. So you must determine what your target market values. Always seeing the same doctor in a group practice? Private rooms and gourmet meals in the hospital? This is information worth knowing.

Research on the Competition

Who are your competitors? What do they offer, and what is the position that they occupy? A unique selling proposition must be just that: unique. You cannot differentiate yourself in the mind of a consumer with a me-too strategy. That said, there may be times when a competitor occupies a space that you want to occupy, and you have reason to think that you can do a better job than the other organization. In that case, your job is to craft the positioning more effectively, get your message out more widely, and live up to your positioning more thoroughly.

Note that your competition may not be immediately obvious. When Scott Cook was starting Intuit, the company that makes the popular accounting software Quicken, he understood that his competition was not other personal finance programs; rather, it was the practice of keeping the household accounts by paper and pencil. In healthcare, the competition may be similar conventional providers or alternative providers. It may be a medical practice in the next county or a hospital in the next state. Alternatively, the competition may be the act of choosing to do without. Many people in the United States do not have health insurance; they put off using the healthcare system as long as they possibly can, and they increasingly engage in self-care.

Operational Assessment

The mission, vision, and values that you have established represent a promise. Keeping that promise means building an organization that lives its values and pursues its mission and vision. Your organization thus has a particular set of capabilities. The position it proposes to occupy, and the reputation it wants to establish, must reflect those capabilities. Put differently, the organization must *execute* consistently and predictably. Wal-Mart cannot promise "everyday low prices" and then be unable to match or best competitors' prices. A hospital cannot promise white-glove treatment of its patients if the staff is not trained to provide it.

Of course, all of these assessments must be made with an eye to the future as well as to the present. Every marketplace is dynamic, and healthcare more than most. How do you expect the marketplace to change? Do you expect new competitors? Can you maintain your operational capabilities over time?

A REPUTATION BASED ON TRUST

To build a trusted reputation, or, more accurately, a reputation based on trust, you must understand the basics of positioning and reputation building. But first, let us turn to the specifics of trust itself—perhaps the most powerful basis for a reputation there is.

The following is a recap of some of the virtues of trust recounted in the early chapters of this book:

- Trust is at the core of all business activity; virtually everthing we do in the business world is carried out by groups of people who have at least a basic trust in one another.
- Without trust, transaction costs rise and transaction time is slowed. Trust thus accelerates the sales/utilization cycle.
- Trust allows people within organizations to work together more effectively. It provides the basis for people to engage in projects and programs that would otherwise be more challenging.
- Trust allows an organization to become an employer of choice. Consumers, suppliers, and referring physicians want to do business with that organization.
- Trust encourages donors to give money and investors to invest money.

In healthcare, trust is essential. In one pharmaceutical company's proprietary study, 94 percent of consumers and 95 percent of healthcare professionals said that trust is either "extremely" or "very" important in the industry. It is the number one predictor of patient loyalty to a physician's practice. In fact, if a consumer or patient does not have a reasonable degree of trust in you to begin with, he or she may never come to see you in the first place. In a recent survey by a faith-based health system, consumers were asked, "What influenced you *most* to use this service?" Reputation and location were tied for first with 25 percent of responses, while physician referral was a close second at 24 percent. In a similar survey by a children's hospital, reputation was the top reason for choosing the hospital. In the *U.S. News & World Report* rankings of America's best hospitals, reputation is one of three variables used to score hospitals, and in some specialties it is the only variable used (Comarow 2004). So powerful is a trusted reputation, in fact, that it leads to absurd survey outcomes. Massachusetts General Hospital, for example, was once ranked as having one of the top ophthalmology programs in the country—even though it has no ophthalmology department. And the Cleveland Clinic was ranked as best in the region for obstetric services, even though, again, it has no obstetrics department.

The initial step, then, is to prepare a positioning promise focused on trust. This does not mean simply coming up with a tagline such as, "The hospital you can trust." Rather, it entails giving people a reason to trust you. Perhaps you can position yourself as the local alternative to big national chains. If you are a faith-based organization, you can play up the importance of your values and ethics (as compared with, say, for-profit competitors). Perhaps you have invested heavily in developing and training a world-class nursing staff and thus can offer a level of nursing care that people cannot find elsewhere. Maybe you offer patients more comprehensive care than your competitors, thanks to your long-term relationships with other providers. Any of these competitive advantages can be the basis for a position based on trust. The point is to draw the connection in the minds of your customers: "You can trust us *because*..."

THE BRAND TOOL KIT

A positioning promise is part of what might be called a "brand tool kit"—a collection of tools and practices that allow an organization to develop and operationalize its positioning and its brand. These are the methods that create the market's identification of the organization in the space it wants to occupy. At a minimum they consist of the copy platform, the elevator speech and slogan, and the positioning guide and graphical standards manual.

Copy Platform

The copy platform describes what you want to sell to your marketplace. In real estate, brokers learn that the most important aspects of any house (after its location) are its curb appeal, its kitchen, and its bathrooms. In healthcare, identifying a copy platform can be more of a challenge. It is not sufficient for a hospital, for example, to say that it has full accreditation, that its physicians are board certified, and that it has the latest technology. These benefits are not unique and are simply regarded as tickets to market entry by consumers. Nor is it sufficient for a managed care organization to say that it has a broad base of physicians and competitive premiums. These, too, are simply tickets to entry.

The key here, again, is to ask yourself why people should trust you and to build a copy platform around the language that describes your advantage. It might be your staff's experience or its training. It might be that you have the friendliest people or that your operations are built around customer convenience. It might be something extra, like an unusual amount of home-based care, or it might simply be an emphasis on consistency of experience ("You know exactly what to expect…"). A copy platform spells out these competitive advantages and relates them to the position focused on trust.

Elevator Speech and Slogan

The "elevator speech"—a 30-second description of the organization's positioning—derives from the copy platform. Its name, of course, comes from the apocryphal ride up the building, in which an elevator companion asks you to describe what your organization does and what is unique about it. The slogan is what might appear on an advertisement, on the wall of your lobby, or on every piece of paper and electronic transmission that leaves the organization.

All of these elements require absolute consistency so that they reinforce the positioning and, in turn, reinforce each other.

Positioning Guide and Graphical Standards Manual

Positioning guides and graphical standards manuals are the brand's "shop manuals"—written notebooks that spell out language to be used (and language to be avoided) in marketing, logos, typefaces, colors, and more. Most large organizations already have them. However, too often they assume that the positioning guide and the graphical standards *are* the positioning and the brand, rather than understanding that they *follow* the positioning and the brand. A brand identity is built around something that is important to the consumer, such as trust. It is not built around a particular logo, color scheme, or slogan. These come last and are chosen to depict your mission, vision, values, and positioning (MV^2P).

IMPLEMENTATION

To put some flesh on the bones of this argument, imagine a regional medical center seeking to build a reputation around trust. The staff of this medical center has been on a six-month-long quest to establish the organization's mission and vision and to codify its values. The journey has revealed the importance of trust to the clinicians and others on the center's staff, and widespread buy-in to the idea of creating an identity based on trust has been achieved.

Now the marketing department conducts extensive research into how consumers perceive this center and its competitors. It finds little or no difference in their perception. It discovers that consumers do not have high amounts of trust in medical organizations in the area. They believe that hospitals are too much concerned with the bottom line. They trust their own doctors, but not doctors as a group; only nurses score high on the trust scale. Like consumers everywhere, they distrust insurance companies, and that distrust spills over into the medical system in general.

So now the brand development operation swings into high gear. The center's senior management determines that its key competitive advantage will lie in care and caring—that is, the actual experience of patients who come into contact with the center. The following operational changes are implemented to support the center's MV^2P and bolster its operational capacity to engender trust:

- The intake process is revamped so that patients are given faster, friendlier service.
- Billing and other financial procedures are changed to allow for maximum transparency.
- Doctors are taking in-house seminars focusing on how they are perceived by patients, and they are coached in techniques that help engender patient trust.
- Other departments are working on improving quality and customer focus.
- A new home care department is created, with a mission of focusing on posthospital follow-up care.
- The nursing service is beefed up through aggressive recruitment of highly skilled nurses.
- Nurses have been provided with free in-house training focusing on the latest techniques of patient care; they have been reorganized into teams, their autonomy boosted, and their pay increased.

The marketing effort communicates the center's key competitive advantage of patients' experience of care and caring and important operations that support these experiences. The copy platform emphasizes the quality of the nursing care, the new home care department, and the caring atmosphere of every department in the hospital. The elevator speech focuses on *why* the care at the center is unique because of new training, fully staffed and up-to-the-minute nursing service, and financial transparency. Two new slogans

What's in a Name?

"What's in a name?" asked Shakespeare's Juliet. "That which we call a rose by any other name would smell as sweet." Name recognition is a key facet of a company's reputation, but it is only one of many. After all, a well-recognized name can by itself be either positive or negative. Enron had great name recognition at the end—but it was recognition that no company would want.

Still, reputation can turn on a name. Whenever Blue Cross–Blue Shield has gone to market with a venture that does *not* carry the organization's name, it has either failed or underperformed. When patients are asked to assess a nameless "hospital" versus an equally nameless "medical center," the hospitals regularly outperform the medical centers. Still, effective branding is not the same as building name recognition or awareness. A company's positioning—its reputation—depends on a host of attributes other than its name.

make their appearance. The tagline "The care you can trust" appears under the center's logo on every bill, every piece of stationery, and every other communication emanating from the hospital. The line "You can trust us to care for *you*" appears on advertisements.

Nurses are made the centerpiece of this effort; they become, in effect, stewards of the brand. Internal communications and ceremonies honor nurses. They are provided with additional training and other perks. The quality of the nursing care receives constant attention from senior management; the nursing staff as a whole is reminded that they are custodians of the center's key mission.

They will also play a role in communicating the brand to the marketplace—a topic to which we now turn in the final chapter.

REFERENCES

Comarow, A. 2004. "Best Hospitals 2004: Methodology." *U.S. News & World Report* [Online article; retrieved 9/22/04.] . http://www.usnews.com/usnews/health/hosptl/methodology.htm.

Sandberg, K. 2002. "Kicking the Tires of Corporate Reputation." *Harvard Management Communication Letter* Jan.: 3.

CHAPTER ELEVEN

Marketing Trust

To be trusted is a greater compliment than to be loved.

—*George MacDonald*

MY PRESCRIPTION FOR trust building in healthcare is outlined in a five-phase approach to the creation, development, and effective utilization of a brand. For convenience and ease of recall, I label each phase with an "R" word; collectively I refer to them as R5, or "R quintic" as it might have once been called. We have already been through the first two phases in this book: establishing your *raison d'être*—your mission, vision, and values—why you exist, where you are going, and the principles that will get you there; and a *reputation*, the position you want to occupy in the marketplace. This chapter is about the three remaining Rs—the three remaining phases of brand strategy and implementation.

Note that the R quintic is a package, as shown in Figure 11.1. None of these phases can be skipped or ignored without compromising the entire approach. Note, too, that it is a sequential process. I have worked with many organizations that plunged right into marketing their brand before they had thought through what they wanted it to stand for in the marketplace and before they had established a mission and vision that were consistent with it. I have also worked with companies that focused so heavily on the mission and vision that they all but forgot about marketing. Neither approach

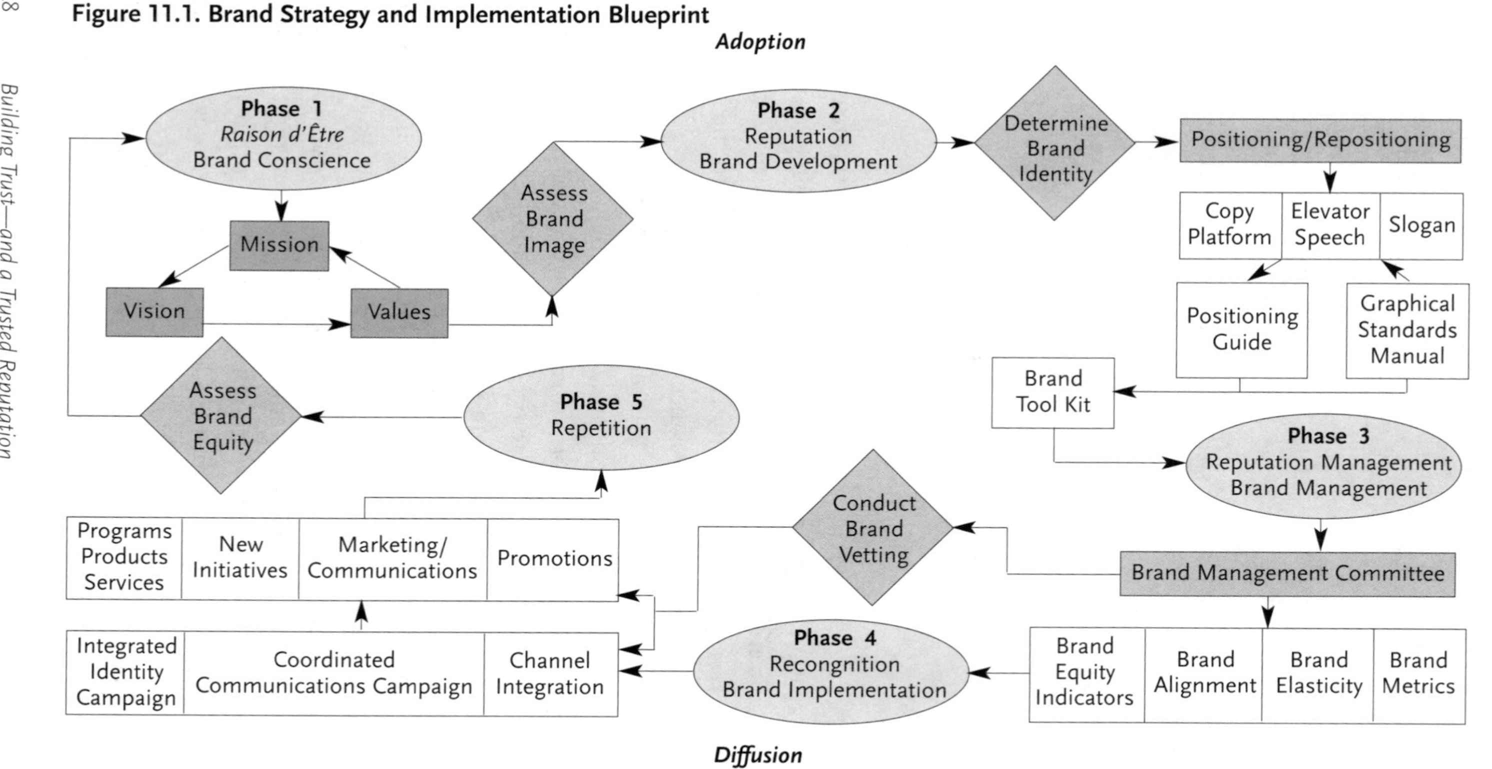

Figure 11.1. Brand Strategy and Implementation Blueprint

Source: ©2005, David A. Shore

is a recipe for success. The five phases are integral to one another; none can be ignored or overlooked.

R3: REPUTATION MANAGEMENT (RELEVANCY TO THE BRAND)

Th reputation management phase—the third—reflects an observation made earlier: Volvo does not make inexpensive cars for 22-year-olds. It does not sponsor NASCAR races. A brand is weakened when a company launches a product or service that does not make sense in light of the brand's positioning. A healthcare organization that is building a brand around trust would be weakened by acquiring a chain of nursing homes that is known for low cost and poor service. A pharmaceutical manufacturer that is asking customers to trust it would be weakened by marketing a line of unproven and possibly harmful nutritional supplements or "natural" remedies. Stated so baldly, the lesson seems obvious, yet companies stretch their brands beyond recognition all the time. The jury is still out, but McDonald's effort to provide more upscale dining in some of its restaurants, complete with fancier décor and a more extensive menu, may prove to be an example of a brand stretched to the breaking point. In healthcare, a comparable stretch is the appearance of concierge or boutique medicine. Concierge or boutique medicine is characterized by the patient paying an additional fee to have better services provided, especially greater access to their physician through off-hours contact and appointments that are longer, guaranteed to occur in the same day scheduled, and prompt (i.e., no waiting for appointments once you arrive). Any organization's move to boutique or concierge medicine should consider its effect on the brand of the organization and also on the healthcare field as a whole. Almost 33 percent of physicians surveyed felt that this type of practice would demean their professional image, and yet 45 percent were in favor of this practice business model (Duke 2004). Time will tell which side will prevail and what the market will prefer.

To ensure that an organization's activities are relevant to its brand and positioning, it needs a high-level, cross-functional reputation management committee. Note the importance of both "high level" and "cross-functional": this group serves a purpose that is far too important to be left to marketing alone. Rather, the committee should be composed of senior managers from a variety of departments. At a minimum, the chief financial officer, chief operating officer, chief information officer, and chief marketing officer should sit on the committee. A healthcare organization should also include the medical director and chief nursing officer, along with other clinical representatives as appropriate. In addition, the committee should involve the people directly charged with communicating with the outside world, in particular the manager responsible for public information or public relations and a representative from any outside advertising or public relations agencies with which the organization works.

The committee's job is at once simple and complex. It is simple because the committee is responsible for one thing and one thing only: the integrity of the brand. In an organization positioned around trust, every single venture that the organization undertakes must be vetted according to whether it builds trust or undermines it. The committee is the enterprise's conscience, and it assesses new ventures and strategies not according to whether they make good business sense but according to how well they contribute to maintaining and developing the brand.

Yet the committee's job is complex because this vetting by brand entails keeping a sharp eye on a variety of metrics and indicators, including brand elasticity, brand metrics, and brand equity.

Brand Elasticity

Every brand can be stretched a certain amount. The catalog company L.L. Bean can offer casual clothing as well as outdoor gear; Jeep can offer a big, four-wheel-drive sport-utility vehicle as well as the traditional army-style vehicle. But there is an obvious limit. L.L. Bean cannot put its name on a chain of office supply stores, and Jeep cannot put its name on a European-style sports car. Exactly where the limits are is a matter of constant debate among marketers and brand managers. Keep your brand too close to home, and you risk passing up good business opportunities; stretch it too far, and the brand becomes meaningless.

Power brands tend to err on the side of caution. Disney is willing to put its name on any product or service that it believes is capable of offering a high-quality entertainment experience ("magic"). Hence there are Disney cruises, Disney theme parks, and the Disney Channel in addition to the company's famous movies. But would any Disney CEO allow the company to lend its name to a travel agency? To a rental car company? How about to an insurance business? Not likely. Similarly, Wal-Mart would not engage in any business that was not conducive to rock-bottom pricing, and the Four Seasons hotel chain would not set up a branded competitor to Motel 6. The companies that own power brands by definition understand how valuable a property they possess, and they are loathe, for very good reason, to test the boundaries of the brand's elasticity.

So it is with a healthcare brand built on trust. Trust is, after all, a highly fragile commodity. It can take years to establish, and it can be destroyed in a remarkably short time. A reputation management committee in this context does well to exercise caution. A new product offering or an acquisition needs to be studied carefully to assess its impact on the brand—and if the impact is likely to be anything but wholly positive, an astute committee will probably find itself deciding to pass on the opportunity. Use the brand elasticity worksheet in Figure 11.2 to evaluate your organization's brand elasticity for specific extensions in relation to your mission, vision, values, and positioning. Simply check the column that represents whether the product/service column is consistent with all of them. Their sum total could be called the "soul of the organization," and opportunities should be measured to see if they are in alignment with the soul

Figure 11.2. Brand Elasticity Worksheet

Product/Service/ Campaign	*Fits*	*Does Not Fit*	*Violates*

of the organization. "Fits" describes alignment. If a community health center's soul involves serving the poor, opening a new clinic in an underserved, economically disadvantaged area is an obvious fit. "Does Not Fit" describes misalignment. If a hospital's soul revolves around caring for patients with illness and injuries, opening a unit for elective cosmetic surgery, while it may be a good business decision, does not align with the purposes of the organization. "Violates" describes extreme misalignment which people find disturbing. If a hospital's soul is to promote health as well as treat illness, and it granted a lease in its food court to a fast food chain notorious for serving unhealthful food, this would violate the soul of the organization. Many people would find that this decision makes them feel worse about the organization, even though they might be doing an excellent job at fulfilling their mission in other areas.

Brand Metrics and Brand Equity

The value of a brand can be measured—not precisely, to be sure, but still with a fair degree of accuracy. Where Coca-Cola is concerned, it could be said that about 90 percent of the company's value lies in its brand and only 10 percent in its other assets. (How much would *you* pay for the Coca-Cola Company, given the proviso that you could not use the name, the distinctive colors and scripts, the advertising themes, or any of the other trappings of the brand?) A company that creates a brand based on trust is creating a valuable asset. That asset must be protected and invested with the same degree of care as any tangible asset.

A variety of metrics guide this process. At any given time, what is the organization's share of the market? What is its share of consumers' minds, as measured by market surveys? What are the attributes and emotions associated with the organization? How likely would consumers be to patronize the organization, to do so more than once, or to recommend it to friends and colleagues? What percentage of customers are repeats, and what percentage are new? All such measures are indications of a brand's equity in the only place it counts: the marketplace.

As the organization contemplates growth—new facilities, new services, acquisitions—the required investment of funds and other resources can be measured against prospective increases (not decreases, one hopes) in the value of the brand. The Mayo Clinic has been able to expand successfully to locations in Arizona and Florida because it was largely able to replicate the high levels of service and expertise provided at its original location in Rochester, Minnesota. The value of this particular power brand was thus maintained and increased. Imagine, by contrast, if Mayo had decided to grow simply by licensing a hundred medical centers around the country to utilize its name. The resulting cheapening of the brand would have undermined decades of building up its value.

R4: RECOGNITION

I call the fourth phase *recognition* for ease of recall, but marketers will understand it as *implementation*, taking your brand to the marketplace.

Marketing is a concept and a function that feels uncomfortable to many healthcare professionals. But this is to mistake the excesses of maketing for its essence. At its root, marketing simply means taking an organization's message—its identity, its capabilities, its offerings—to the people it is trying to serve. If the organization's mission is worthwhile, as it usually is in healthcare, then marketing that mission is worthwhile as well. How else can the people who might utilize an organization's services learn about it? So I will ask you to set aside whatever prejudices you may have about marketing and consider the sequence of steps that make for an effective brand recognition effort.

The heart of such an effort is a *coordinated, integrated identity campaign.* In other words, do not begin with an advertising campaign, a promotion, or the introduction of a new service. Consider as a whole the positioning promise you have crafted and the brand identity you have decided to establish. Your goal now is to establish this space in the marketplace, to reinforce it at every opportunity, and to make it yours. Remember Volvo's approach: the safety emphasis on its web site; the slogan ("For life") appearing on every advertisement; even the thick, durable feel of its brochures—everything reinforces the image of safety. So should it be with trust, if that is to be your organization's centerpiece. The language and images of trust should permeate every aspect of every form of communication, from the tagline on stationery to the décor on the office or clinic walls. Colors and typefaces should be chosen to reinforce trust. This is indeed possible; ask any competent designer for guidance.

Once such an identity campaign has been created—once the parameters and the language are in place—the many tools of marketing can be put to effective use.

Communications Campaigns

The quickest way to get your message out is to package it in appealing stories and take it to the public through the media and other channels. This is sometimes called public relations—again, a phrase that is difficult for many healthcare professionals to accept—but it might just as well be called public information. What steps has your organization taken to make itself more trustworthy? What examples can you point to that show your commitment to building trust? What stories can you tell about your positive impact on patients, your staff, and the community as a whole?

The point here is to turn the trust famine to your advantage. It is not news that consumers mistrust healthcare organizations. But what if a healthcare provider acknowledges the trust famine, takes concrete steps to address the lack of trust, and commits itself to becoming the one organization in its marketplace that consumers *can* trust? In the case of our hypothetical medical center, a commitment to building up a world-class nursing service ("the care you can trust"), complete with pay raises, training programs, and the other accouterments of quality, instantly sets the center apart from competitors with short-staffed and overworked nursing services. This will be news, and communicating it will attract the attention of both the media and the community.

Marketing Communications

The traditional vehicles of marketing communications—literature and brochures, advertising, a web site, educational materials—can also be put to effective use in building trust. This is not just a matter of attaching the appropriate slogans to every piece, though that is an essential step. It is primarily a matter of highlighting what the organization is doing to build a trustworthy environment. Why not tell the world exactly how the organization is revamping its financial procedures to encourage greater transparency? Why not tell the world that its physicians are committed to earning the trust of their patients, and exactly how they are going about it? Too often, ads and other communications vehicles focus on what might be termed generic benefits, that is, benefits to which any competing organization could lay equal claim. Effective marketing communications focus on unique benefits. A commitment to building trust is just such a benefit.

There is another huge opportunity for building trust through marketing communications. Most marketing campaigns are a one-way street: an organization prints up its literature and commissions its advertising, yet makes no allowance for feedback from the people it is trying to reach. Imagine, then, the effect of an organization that regularly asks for input and actually pays attention to the input it receives. "We want to earn your trust: tell us how!" would be one of the most powerful statements any organization could make. Every piece of literature and every advertisement should contain an e-mail address and a telephone number for consumer response. The web site should be designed to encourage and facilitate interactive communication (a potential of this medium that nearly every company has so far left unrealized). One major trust-buster in healthcare is the simple fact that consumers feel powerless to express their concerns to busy physicians and faceless institutions. Opening up authentic and responsive two-way channels of communication is thus an almost automatic trust builder.

Promotions

Promotions are necessarily different in healthcare than in other industries. You can hardly advertise a special on echocardiograms ("This month only!") or give people a $50 coupon for switching to your HMO. But well-conceived promotions are no less effective for being different. A stop-smoking campaign, an educational campaign about breast cancer or another disease, and sponsorship of a walkathon for physical fitness are all efforts that draw favorable attention to a healthcare organization and hence can be an important part of its marketing. Promotions focusing on trust can be equally effective and engaging. Suppose a nursing home were to sponsor a scrupulously honest educational campaign on the pluses and minuses of long-term-care insurance, complete with outreach into the community. Suppose an insurance company developed a "Get a Checkup!" campaign and paid for the checkup regardless of whether the patient had a policy with that company (or, indeed, whether the patient had any insurance at all). Suppose a hospital put a section entitled "How to read a hospital bill" on its web site and showed patients how transparent and easy it is to understand its bills. These are promotions, no less so than the $1.69 special at the supermarket, but they are promotions that are appropriate to healthcare. They are also promotions appropriate to building trust.

New Initiatives

Just as marketing is part and parcel of what the organization is and does, so are its new initiatives a part of its marketing. New initiatives include such efforts as the following:

- A new product or service offering, such as an insurance plan tailored to seniors
- A revamped medical facility, such as a newly equipped radiology lab
- An acquisition, such as the purchase of a nursing home in a nearby community
- A process or procedural improvement, such as new intake and billing procedures
- A new medical focus, such as an emphasis on sports medicine

Healthcare organizations, like most companies, often view such initiatives opportunistically; that is, they create something new when the opportunity arises. What I am proposing is that they regard new initiatives not opportunistically but strategically. What is missing in our trust portfolio? How would a new initiative in this or that arena contribute to building our brand as a trusted organization? These questions, rather than return on investment or any other opportunistic guideline, should drive the organization's decision, and the brand management committee should be heavily involved in making that decision.

Over time, new initiatives become part of the organization's lineup of programs, products, and services. The organization's offerings to the marketplace are dynamic and hence present an opportunity to focus on the trust builders and discard the trustbusters.

R5: REPETITION

There is one more step to the R quintic brand development model, R5, which is repetition. Organizations that seek to develop power brands cannot do it in a quarter or even in a year. It is a commitment that lasts year after year after year, and it is based on taking the same message to the marketplace over and over and over throughout all touch points. Part of the reason that repetition is necessary, of course, is that it takes messages a while to sink in. When people hear the same thing from an organization over time, they begin to associate that message with the organization, to test it out, and, if it passes the test, to accept it. But another part of the reason is that consistency itself is a hallmark of trust. Trust is not simply this year's fad; it is not a marketing campaign (in the Madison Avenue sense) that will be here today and gone tomorrow. An organization that builds an identity based on trust is building an identity for the ages, and it behooves that organization never to stray one iota from its emphasis on trust. Repetition of the message signifies consistency of commitment.

ASSESSING BRAND EQUITY

I have said that the brand development model is a five-phase sequential model, and so it is. But it is also circular. The creation of a *raison d'être* or brand conscience—a mission, vision, and set of values based on trust—leads to brand development, the point at which brand identity and reputation are established. Brand management (relevancy) takes this creation and manages it as it goes to the marketplace, earning recognition. The message is repeated over time until it is firmly established.

But this is not a once-and-for-all process. Once the brand has been taken to the marketplace, once the messages have been crafted and implemented, it is time again to assess the brand's equity and judge its consistency with the organization's mission, vision, and values. Nothing in healthcare—indeed, nothing anywhere in the world these days—is static. So the organization must ask itself whether what it has done is consistent with its *raison d'être* and whether anything in the environment has changed so that the implementation of the brand's identity must be modified. Mission, vision, and values (MV^2) do not change, or if they do, they evolve only gradually, over decades. But the identity and messages that are based on this MV^2 may appear somewhat different from one year to the next. Trust, of course, is a constant. But *how* the organization focuses on building trust can change, just because people's perceptions of what they do and do not trust are likely to change.

REFERENCE

Duke, A. 2004. "Doctors Give Mixed Reviews to Boutique Medicine." *Access News*. [Online article; retrieved 9/24/04.] http://www.axcessnews.com/health_080804.shtml.

Epilog

A TRUST INITIATIVE

A number of years ago I delivered the keynote address at the *Wall Street Journal* Health Care Summit. My topic was building a power brand in healthcare. At the end of the lecture, I added extemporaneously, "The healthcare brand that owns trust owns its marketplace," and asked, "After all, can you think of something that you would rather be known for than to be a trusted provider of high-quality goods and services?" I had recently identified the importance of trust while doing brand diagnostics for healthcare organizations, and the *Wall Street Journal* summit was the perfect venue to launch a trial balloon to test the value of trust diagnostics. These healthcare industry leaders responded better than I could have hoped, nodding attentively in agreement with my statement and peppering me with questions and comments afterward. Many said that they had never before been conscious of this issue as it applied to themselves and their organizations, and they enthusiastically expressed their interest. Such a high level of interest expressed by these key industry decision makers impelled me to pursue the topic further.

I began to filter my experience on this day through a lens of trust, which allowed me to identify the fundamental issues of trust appearing again and again in the events that became the healthcare headlines. Thus, I expanded my work to include trust equity in addition to brand equity. I began to examine the return on investment of trust and to conduct not only brand diagnostics but also trust diagnostics. Branding is fundamentally about having a reputation with distinction in the marketplace. In working with organizations on branding, time and again I came to the same conclusion: just about no one in the healthcare market owned trust. In keeping with the Socratic tradition, after completing a competitive analysis of an organization, I would ask the question of the leadership team, "If you were to decide you wanted to build your brand around trust, who would be your competition?" The answer almost universally was, "We would have no competition." So the problem in a nutshell was that the demand for more trusted providers (and employers) is great, whereas the supply is scare, but this problem is also a great opportunity for forward-thinking healthcare leaders.

In the past five years, as I have continued to research trust in healthcare and business, I have been struck by its universal significance. An MBA graduate told me in wonderment that she had never touched on the topic of trust in her studies, yet found it one of the most vital issues in her work now that she was conscious of it. A cancer patient identified trust as the main way he made decisions in choosing his providers, regimens, and institutions. A physician executive identified trust as integral to doing his job as both a pediatrician and as a hospital medical director. A surgeon reflected on how a patient must feel, after having met her for only a few minutes with no time to develop familiarity or intimacy to then trust her, literally, with his life. Virtually everyone is touched by issues of trust, be they purchasers, payers, suppliers, hospitals, employees, physicians, or patients.

My colleagues at the Harvard School of Public Health and elsewhere in the university agreed when I sought out their opinion on whether the topic of trust was worthy of institutionalizing. And so the Trust Initiative was established at the Harvard School of Public Health with the enthusiastic support of the school's leadership and the generous academic support of my colleagues.

Given that trust always has been important and always will be important, I expect that the research and teaching on trust conducted by myself and others will continue to yield valuable insight and contributions. I hope this book has stimulated your interest and shown you how to use the power of trust to improve your organization's mission and margin, as well as improve our troubled healthcare system.